T0202212

In Defense of the
Human Being

In Defense of the Human Being
Foundational Questions of an Embodied Anthropology

Thomas Fuchs

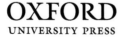

OXFORD
UNIVERSITY PRESS

OXFORD

UNIVERSITY PRESS

Great Clarendon Street, Oxford, OX2 6DP,
United Kingdom

Oxford University Press is a department of the University of Oxford.
It furthers the University's objective of excellence in research, scholarship,
and education by publishing worldwide. Oxford is a registered trade mark of
Oxford University Press in the UK and in certain other countries

© Suhrkamp Verlag 2021

The moral rights of the author have been asserted

First Edition published in 2021

Impression: 6

Published in the United States of America by Oxford University Press
198 Madison Avenue, New York, NY 10016, United States of America

British Library Cataloguing in Publication Data

Data available

Library of Congress Control Number: 2021935956

ISBN 978-0-19-289819-7

DOI: 10.1093/oso/9780192898197.001.0001

Printed and bound by
CPI Group (UK) Ltd, Croydon, CR0 4YY

With the progress of artificial intelligence, the digitalization of the life-world, and the reduction of the mind to neuronal processes, the human being appears more and more as a product of data and algorithms. We understand ourselves in the image of our machines, while conversely, we elevate our machines and our brains to new subjects. Against this self-reification of the human being, the philosopher and psychiatrist Thomas Fuchs defends a humanism of embodiment: our corporeality, vitality, and embodied freedom are the foundations of a self-determined existence that uses the new technologies as means instead of submitting to them.

Thomas Fuchs, psychiatrist and philosopher, is Karl Jaspers Professor for Philosophical Foundations of Psychiatry at Heidelberg University and chairs the research section "Phenomenological Psychopathology and Psychotherapy" at the Psychiatric University Hospital Heidelberg.

Contents

B Brain, Person, and Reality

4 Person and Brain: Against Cerebrocentrism *107*

5 Embodied Freedom: A Libertarian Position *124*

Abbreviations

AI   artificial intelligence
AL   artificial life

Introduction: A Humanism of Embodiment

The image of the human being that we hold to be true becomes itself a factor in our lives. It determines the ways in which we deal with ourselves and with other people, it determines our attitude in life and our choice of tasks.

Karl Jaspers (1948: 56)

In Defense of the Human Being—this title requires explanation. A defense can be directed against a criticism or accusation, but also against a questioning or a threat. Now, there is a long tradition of putting humanity itself in the dock, accusing humans of immoderateness, greed, hubris, or malice, for the horrors of war or the destruction of the planet. Recently, there have even been many suggestions that it would be best for the planet if it could free itself from its "mold," as Schopenhauer once called humanity.[1] Homo sapiens has abused its supremacy, so the argument runs, and therefore deserves to perish by a collapse of the ecosystem or other catastrophes—or to make way for a superior artificial super-intelligence. At a moment when geologists have already proclaimed the new planetary age of the *Anthropocene* to describe the comprehensive transformation of the Earth by humans, some argue that it would be better if this age were the shortest of all.[2]

----

[1] In infinite space countless shining spheres, around every one of them rotate perhaps a dozen illuminated smaller ones, hot within, covered with a solidified, cold rind, on which a moldy covering has produced living and knowing beings:—that is the empirical truth, the real, the world (Schopenhauer 1859/1966: 3).

[2] Humanity as the "plague of the planet" is a *topos* particularly of radical ecological movements; for example, the Voluntary Human Extinction Movement, founded in 1991

In Defense of the Human Being. Thomas Fuchs, Oxford University Press. © Suhrkamp Verlag 2021.
DOI: 10.1093/oso/9780192898197.003.0001

An apology for humanity against such misanthropy might be appropriate, but it is not my theme. It is not my concern to defend humanity against an accusation, but against a *questioning*. Because today, in question is what one could call—with unavoidable imprecision—the humanistic image of man. At the center of this image is the human person as a physical or embodied being, as a free, self-determining being, and ultimately as an essentially social being connected with others. According to this understanding, persons are not mere spirits or monads of consciousness but embodied, living beings. And persons do not exist in the singular but only in a common relational space. In the concept of human dignity, understood as the claim to recognition that human beings raise through their bodily existence and co-existence, the definitions that constitute a humanistic, personal image of humanity culminate and unite.[3] To what extent is this self-image of man currently in question?

Beyond Freedom and Dignity is the title of a book published in 1971 by B. F. Skinner, an American behavioral psychologist. Skinner argued that belief in something like free will and moral autonomy was the relic of a mythical, prescientific view of man. The attribution of personal responsibility and dignity impedes scientific progress on its way to conditioning human behavior through appropriate social technology and thus creating a happier society without overpopulation and wars. Skinner's behaviorist vision has failed to take hold. But his basic idea that science is capable of replacing our self-conception, which is caught up in prejudice and myth, with a rational knowledge of human beings, and with corresponding technologies is more relevant than ever.

In his book *Homo Deus* (2017), the historian Yuval Noah Harari has sketched out a gloomy scenario for the future, according to which scientific and technological progress will gradually render the liberal and humanistic view of humanity obsolete. According to Harari, we will increasingly surrender to the

----

by Les Knight, advocates the extinction of humanity to save the Earth (cf. their website www.vhemt.org). Robert Ettinger has drawn another, specifically transhumanistic conclusion:

> Thus, humanity itself is a disease, of which we must now proceed to cure ourselves […]. To do this, it must first be shown that homo sapiens is only a botched beginning; when he clearly sees himself as an error, he may not only be motivated to sculpt himself, but to make at least a few swift and confident strokes. (Ettinger 1989: 4, 8f.)

[3] Of course, representatives of transhumanism also refer to a "secular humanism" (for example, Bostrom 2005: 202). But, in this interpretation, the term is decoupled from its classical tradition, which goes back to the Renaissance, and is used to designate decidedly atheistic positions that often connect with a reductive naturalism too.

algorithms,[4] data analyses, and forecasts of artificial intelligence, as they can already provide better information about the future than our limited human intelligence:

> People will no longer see themselves as autonomous beings running their lives according to their wishes, but instead will become accustomed to seeing themselves as a collection of biochemical mechanisms that is constantly monitored and guided by a network of electronic algorithms. (Harari 2017: 334)

Harari, with constant recourse to the biological and cybernetic sciences, and having thoroughly destroyed the foundations of the liberal view of man, nevertheless wants to leave open the possibility that science could be wrong after all: "Is there perhaps something in the universe that cannot be reduced to data?" (Harari 2017: 399). "Are organisms really just algorithms and is life really just data processing?" (Harari 2017: 402). If not, says Harari, then perhaps something could be lost after all if people let themselves be controlled (and in the end even be replaced) by intelligent machines. But after all Harari's fatalistic remarks this is no more than a *façon de parler*. For him it remains the case that "*Homo sapiens* is an obsolete algorithm" (Harari 2017: 381).

Now it is beyond doubt that the sort of view of humans Harari depicts can have very real consequences. In China, we are currently seeing how an authoritarian regime is establishing a digital surveillance apparatus by means of artificial intelligence. A "social credit system" records and evaluates the consumption and relationship preferences of citizens, their political and social behavior, their creditworthiness and conformity, right down to their criminal record. Facial recognition software, which evaluates public video surveillance, can easily be linked to the system. This is where something like Skinner's social technology is now being realized and digital dystopias are taking shape.

Nevertheless, defending the human being, his freedom and dignity, must not be limited to painting a gloomy picture of the future. Rather, it must be about criticizing the assumptions behind a *scientistic view of humans*, which authors like Harari uncritically adopt. These assumptions include in particular the following:

- *Naturalism*: from the point of view of reductionist naturalism, there are no phenomena that elude a complete scientific explanation. In particular, subjectivity, mind, and consciousness can be traced back to physical or

---

[4] Algorithms can be described in simplified terms as defined chains of events with which a system reacts to an input, for example according to the rule: "if a, then b"—"if not a, then c." Algorithms form the basic structure of the programs which computers run.

physiological processes, i.e., they can be regarded as products of determined neuronal processes. They have no independent effectiveness in the world.

- *Elimination of the living*: the biosciences regard organisms in principle as biological machines controlled by genetic programs. Selfhood, experience or subjectivity no longer appear in this paradigm. The fact that a cat hunts a mouse can then be explained as the effect of biochemical or evolutionary mechanisms—taking its hunger or hunting instinct as a basis is now considered a naive anthropomorphism.

- *Functionalism*: phenomena of consciousness are attributed to processes of neuronal information processing, which transform an input into a suitable output according to algorithmic rules. In principle, these digital processes can run on any carrier ("hardware"), and they can even be simulated by artificial systems. Because it is not the subjective experience but only the function, i.e., data processing and the corresponding output, that constitutes the mind.

If these interlinked assumptions were correct, then humans would be far better understood in terms of neuronal processes, genetic algorithms, and digitized behavioral patterns, in short, as the sum of their data, than through hermeneutical understanding, self-reflection, and self-awareness. The "know thyself" of the Delphic oracle would be outdated—the Google algorithms would know us better. The modern chorus of materialistic neuro-philosophy proclaims that our subjective experience is nothing more than the colorful "user interface of a neuro-computer and thus a user illusion" (Slaby 2011)—only the neuronal computational processes in the background are real. From this point of view, subjectivity, self-awareness, and self-determination become epiphenomena which, in everyday life we may still believe in, but which to regard as reality only testifies to naivety and nostalgia.

A defense of the humanistic view of humans, as undertaken in this volume, would be ill-advised if it were limited to proving that consciousness and subjectivity are irreducible. Such a defense would only follow pre-determined dualistic paths—here mind, there body, here qualitative inwardness, there measurable objective facts. In view of the progress of neurobiology, but also in view of increasing digitalization and virtualization, such a defense of a "citadel of the subject"[5] could soon prove ineffective—especially if subjectivity and its expressions become *simulated* more and more convincingly. It is not inconceivable that the simulation of human by artificial intelligence and the simulation of physical presence by robots or virtual avatars could increasingly take the place of human reality. When, for example, do we begin to ascribe something like

---

[5] On this, see Fuchs 2018: xvi–xx.

consciousness to Alexa or Siri on the basis that they express their feelings so convincingly and understand our own feelings so well?

This brings me to the subtitle of the volume, "Embodied Anthropology." According to my thesis, the actual alternative to a naturalistic-reductive image of the human being consists in attention to the *embodiment and aliveness*[6] that are constitutive of the person. No abstract inwardness, disembodied consciousness or pure spirit are the guiding ideas of a humanistic view of the person, but the person's concrete physical existence. Only when it can be shown that the person is present in his body itself, that the person feels, perceives, expresses, and acts with his whole body, do we escape confinement in a hidden inner space of consciousness, an inaccessible citadel from which only signals penetrate to the outside world, signals which can no longer be distinguished from the those of an artificial intelligence. And, only when persons have an embodied freedom, i.e., determine themselves *as organisms* in decisions and actions, does subjectivity become more than an epiphenomenon, i.e., *really effective* in the world.

Only as embodied, physical beings are we real for each other too. There is no communication or empathy between brains, even if neuroscientists like to claim that.[7] We only learn empathy through physical contact with other persons, through "intercorporeality," as Merleau-Ponty called it. And we understand others primarily not through a "theory of mind," as current developmental psychology assumes, but already intuitively through the other's bodily expressions, gestures, and behavior. Only a few weeks after birth, babies recognize the emotional expressions of the mother or father, namely by understanding and feeling these expressions' melody, rhythm, and dynamics in their own bodies. *Theories* about the inner life of others only need to be formed by autistic people who have not developed this social intuition—so to say, the *musical sense* for the resonances of intercorporeality—from birth onwards.[8]

One might object that we are increasingly moving and communicating in virtual spaces, where our embodiment is becoming more and more obsolete. Recently, the Covid-19 pandemic has furthered the disembodiment of our social life and seems to be triggering a new digitalization push. In the face of global digital networking, human corporeality can increasingly appear as an atavism, from which transhumanists would like to free us through *mind uploading*.[9]

---

[6] The rather unusual term "aliveness" is used in the following to describe the condition of being alive or a living organism; "vitality" has more the connotation of vigor or joy of life.

[7] See, for example, De Vignemont and Singer (2006); or Hein and Singer (2008).

[8] On this, see Fuchs and De Jaegher (2009); and Fuchs (2015).

[9] See Chapter 2 "Beyond the Human?" in this volume.

However, apart from the fact that the sentient body is very much a part of any virtual spaces—as every excitement while watching a movie testifies—every digitally mediated online communication presupposes that, beyond all mediation, we are still dealing with a living human being of flesh and blood.[10] In other words, all online communication has as its starting or end point the *concrete, physical encounter*. Even in a primarily virtual interaction we always anticipate this encounter, at least as a possibility.

What the present defense is based on, then, is less the classical humanism of the spirit than a *humanism of the living, embodied spirit*. As such, it makes use not only of philosophical (in particular phenomenological) analysis but also of the concepts of *embodiment, extended mind*, and *enactive cognition*, which have become increasingly important in recent years.[11] The fact that humans are not dualistically divided beings of mind and body but above all a living beings of flesh and blood, and as such simultaneously experiencing and aware of themselves—this insight, already found in Aristotle and which today needs to be revived, will form the guiding thread of the following essays. The concepts mentioned previously not only allow for a critical analysis of current scientific and technological developments but also for their productive integration without falling into a backward-looking cultural pessimism. In this sense, the present defense of the human being can certainly be seen as a "defense forward"—namely toward a new, embodied anthropology. Even an ecological redefinition of our relationship to the earthly environment will only succeed if our corporeality and aliveness—as connectedness or *conviviality* with our natural environment—is at its center. Only if we inhabit our bodies will we also be able to maintain the earth in a habitable form.

The texts collected here, written in recent years and with a view to such an embodied anthropology, explore, in particular, the following topics:

- The *progress of artificial intelligence and robotics* is increasingly challenging the distinction between simulation and the reality of the human being. They suggest on the one hand a computeromorphic understanding of human intelligence, on the other hand an anthropomorphization of artificial intelligence (AI) systems. In other words: we are seeing ourselves more and more like our machines and vice versa. So, what distinguishes human and artificial intelligence? And does the essence of the human being consist of information?

---

[10] See Chapter 3 "The Virtual Other" in this volume.

[11] See, for example, Varela et al. (1991); Thompson (2007); Fingerhut et al. (2013); and Fuchs (2018).

- *Transhumanism* regards the human in its present state of development as basically imperfect. The result of evolution is only a blindly grown and therefore poorly constructed, defective product. Our goal should be to create a "Homo optimus" or to free our mind completely from the biological body. Is there a meaningful concept of the posthuman?

- The increasing spread of *virtuality and digital media* also tends to cancel out the difference between embodiment and simulation. When the "virtual other" takes the place of real encounters it becomes all the more important to analyze the potentials and limits of virtual worlds. What distinguishes real and virtual encounters?

- Advances in the *neurosciences* have been instrumental in making human subjectivity appear as an epiphenomenon of brain processes and in undermining the idea of personal freedom. So, are we just creatures of our neurons? Concepts of embodied subjectivity and embodied freedom are able to correct such reductionist views.

- Closely linked to the developments mentioned so far is the widespread thesis of *constructivism*, according to which our perception is no more than an illusory and deceptive construction of subjective realities. This thesis undermines our primary trust in the shared world and fosters the tendencies toward virtualization. How can perception be rehabilitated as an intersubjective constitution of reality?

- In *psychiatry*, naturalistic concepts have led to a reductionist, "cerebrocentric" view of mental illness, which does not do justice to the patients' experiences and relationships. Does mental suffering really exhaust itself in brain processes? Such views can be contrasted with an embodied and ecological view of the psyche, which can provide a new foundation for psychiatry as *relational medicine*.

- *Acceleration and digitalization processes* finally lead, in western societies, to a repression of the cyclical, bodily rhythms of human time in favor of the monolinear time of growth and acceleration, with well-known psychological and ecological consequences such as burn-out and climate change. To what extent does embodied, lived time resist its socialization and acceleration? These forms and conflicts of temporality must be analyzed in order to better understand social dynamics and to develop strategies for balancing cyclical and linear time.

The most important themes of the following essays are thus identified. It is to be hoped that they will achieve their goal of contributing to the defense of the human—not least against humanity's own voluntarism. Because modernity's endeavor to "transform everything given into something made"—as Gernot

Böhme (2010: 143) aptly puts it—has today reached a point where the constitution and freedom of the human being itself is called into question. And it will not only be a question of theoretical reason but an ethical and ultimately a political question whether in this situation a humanistic view of the human being can be defended and at the same time redefined. For, as Karl Jaspers wrote, the image of the human being that we consider to be true ultimately determines how we deal with ourselves and with others—today, we should add: and with nature. Humanism in the ethical sense therefore means resistance to the rule and constraints of technocratic systems as well as to the self-reification and mechanization of humans. If we conceive of ourselves as objects, be it as algorithms or as neuronally determined apparatuses, then we surrender ourselves to the rule of those who seek to manipulate such apparatuses and to control them socio-technologically. "For the power of Man to make himself what he pleases means [...] the power of some men to make other men what *they* please" (Lewis 1943/2009: 59). The defense of man is, in this respect, not only a theoretical task but also an ethical duty.

Acknowledgments

I would like to thank Adrian Wilding for his invaluable help with the translation. During the production process I was happy to collaborate with Jade Dixon and Martin Baum from Oxford University Press and with Madhanraj Tharanendran from Newgen Knowledge Works who provided all necessary support.

References

Böhme, G. 2010. "Das Gegebene und das Gemachte." In M. Großheim and S. Kluck (eds.) *Phänomenologie und Kulturkritik. Über die Grenzen der Quantifizierung*. Freiburg: Alber (pp. 140–50).

Bostrom, N. 2005. "In defense of posthuman dignity." *Bioethics* 19: 202–14.

de Vignemont, F., T. Singer. 2006. "The empathic brain: How, when and why?" *Trends in Cognitive Sciences* 10: 435–41.

Ettinger, R. C. 1989. *Man into Superman*. New York: Avon.

Fingerhut, J., R. Hufendiek, M. Wild (ed.). 2013. *Philosophie der Verkörperung. Grundlagentexte zu einer aktuellen Debatte*. Berlin: Suhrkamp.

Fuchs, T. 2015. "Pathologies of intersubjectivity in autism and schizophrenia." *Journal of Consciousness Studies* 22: 191–214.

Fuchs, T. 2018. *Ecology of the Brain: The Phenomenology and Biology of the Embodied Mind*. Oxford: Oxford University Pres.

Fuchs, T., H. De Jaegher. 2009. "Enactive intersubjectivity: Participatory sense-making and mutual incorporation." *Phenomenology and the Cognitive Sciences* 8: 465–86.

Harari, Y. N. 2017. *Homo Deus: A Brief History of Tomorrow*. New York: Harper.

Hein, G., T. Singer. 2008. "I feel how you feel but not always: The empathic brain and its modulation." *Current Opinion in Neurobiology* 18: 153–8.

Jaspers, K. 1948. *Der philosophische Glaube*. Zürich: Artemis.

Lewis, C. S. 2009. *The Abolition of Man*. New York: Harper (First published 1943).

Schopenhauer, A. 1966. *The World as Will and Representation*, 2 vols., E. F. J. Payne (trans.) New York: Dover (First published 1859).

Skinner, B. F. 1971. *Beyond Freedom and Dignity*. New York: Bantam Books.

Slaby, J. 2011. "Perspektiven einer kritischen Philosophie der Neurowissenschaften." *Deutsche Zeitschrift für Philosophie* 59: 375–90.

Thompson, E. 2007. *Mind in Life. Biology, Phenomenology, and the Sciences of Mind*. Cambridge, MA: Harvard University Press.

Varela, F. J., E. Thompson, E. Rosch. 1991. *The Embodied Mind: Cognitive Science and Human Experience*. Cambridge, MA: MIT Press.

A

Artificial Intelligence, Transhumanism, Virtuality

Chapter 1

Human and Artificial Intelligence: A Clarification

Where is the wisdom we have lost in knowledge?
Where is the knowledge we have lost in information?

T. S. Eliot (1934)

Introduction: The World of Data

With the technological developments of the present age, we are witnessing an astonishing dematerialization. Never before in history has the disembodiment of the spirit, the sublimation of matter into a pure form, the transformation of everything physical into numbers and signs reached such a scale as it does today. Data streams orbit the globe at the speed of light, digital algorithms create virtual realities, and intelligent robots operate factories. The world of finance is decoupling itself from the real production of goods in ever more sublimated derivatives, and stock trading is largely conducted by computer systems. Knowledge is detached from knowing subjects, digitalized, and transformed into the electrical oscillations of the clouds, quantified in mega-, giga- and terabytes. Artificial intelligence (AI) is beginning to learn and is already surpassing the first achievements of human intelligence. Indeed, the subjective mind itself appears in the end only as a sum of algorithms, a complex data structure in the brain, which in principle could also be realized by other data carriers and is no longer bound to the earthly physical body.

At first glance, this seems to be a paradox. After all, materialism or physicalism, at least in Western culture, represents the predominant world view. No one refers these days to immaterial souls, etheric forces, or divine influences unless he wants to receive—at best—an indulgent smile. But the dematerialization of matter is today proceeding in different terms. The magic word of the spirit is *information*. Originally meaning *a message for someone*, information has come to mean independent, freely convertible data, signals, and codes, movable and volatile, available for arbitrary access, and only incidentally bound

In Defense of the Human Being. Thomas Fuchs, Oxford University Press. © Suhrkamp Verlag 2021.
DOI: 10.1093/oso/9780192898197.003.0002

to any material carrier. On the wings of electromagnetic energy and at the speed of light, the spirit has escaped the inertia of matter as far as possible.

The world today seems to be filled with information, indeed, to literally *consist of information*: "messenger molecules" are able to "read" the alphabet of the genome and to pass on its information; receptors and nerves supply the brain with information, which is then processed in neuronal networks to form the mind, while outside in electronic networks information circulates freely around the world. As early as the mid-1950s, Carl Friedrich von Weizsäcker developed the theory that matter and energy originate from information, i.e., from "0" and "1" as binary primordial elements. Though information is insubstantial, scientists "wonder whether it may be primary: more fundamental than matter itself" (Gleick 2011: 10). Some physicists now describe the entire universe as a quantum computer, a cosmic information processing machine, and its history as a gigantic quantum bit calculation: "Whatever is happening in the universe […] is all information" (Paul & Cox 1996: 34).

Where everything thus seems to consist of pieces of information, each informing the other, a simple truth is all too easily overlooked: information only exists *where someone understands something*—that is, news *as news*, signs *as signs*. Information exists only for conscious living beings, or for persons.[1] The encoding of messages as data and their transfer to a carrier medium does not generate information that would pertain to the carrier as such but at best *potential* information which only becomes *actual* information when decoded by a person. Nor does a computer contain any "information": it "computes" only from the user's point of view—considered in isolation, the apparatus merely converts electronic patterns into other patterns according to programmed algorithms. Only the output of the apparatus—for example, a printout or what is visible on the screen—can be understood once again by the user. An "information-processing system" can therefore only ever be spoken of from the perspective of *a person who interprets the system as such*.[2] The transfer of the concept of information to natural objects such as genes or neuron activities,

---

[1] Of course, a pseudo concept of information originating in communications engineering has become widespread today, a concept deprived of any meaning and expressed quantitatively in "bits"—see the following section.

[2] "The problem with the concept of 'information processing' is that information processing is typically in the mind of an observer. For example, we treat a computer as a processor and a bearer of information, but intrinsically, the computer is only an electronic circuit. […] The electrical state transitions of a computer are symbol manipulations only relative to the attachment of a symbolic interpretation by some designer, programmer, or user" (Searle 1998: 1941).

which were not created and programmed for human purposes, becomes even more problematic. And a universe of information, which would not be understood by anyone, would be—if one does not call on God to help—a meaningless term.

Nevertheless, talking about "genetic information" or "information processing in the brain" has become so ubiquitous that it almost seems futile to question it (for a critique, see Janich 2018). However, at least in scientific theory, we should be aware that we are only dealing here with metaphors. Giving up the (inter-) subjectivity of information would indeed render the notion completely arbitrary: why shouldn't even an oxygen molecule contain "information" that is transferred to other molecules, which, depending on their own "information processing," associate with the former or just move on? But obviously, the term information *would not add anything to the causal explanation* which we can give of an oxygen reaction. On the contrary, it would introduce a new entity which must itself be explained, and we would be well advised to apply Occam's razor to it.[3]

This leads to another important consequence: if consciousness is necessary to understand information, that is, to see something like information in the structures and patterns of the world in the first place, then it cannot itself consist of information. As conscious beings we are "informed," i.e., we have knowledge, expertise, and information. But the consciousness of all this information *is not itself yet more information*. Because this information would have to be understood by another consciousness in order to be information, namely by a consciousness that would itself be information again, and so on, i.e., an infinite regress. Consciousness itself cannot be composed of information.

But there is also no homunculus in the brain that is able to decipher any information about the world from neuronal activity patterns. The brain as such does not possess any information. Undoubtedly, neuronal signal processing and pattern formation in the brain are necessary *for us* to be able to absorb and understand information—but we still have to do this ourselves, our brain cannot do it for us. It is only a necessary condition for this. Information is only available where *someone understands something*, and that is the person, not their brain.

---

[3] See also Manzotti & Owcarz (2020). This has not stopped information scientists from using the term as if denoting existing facts; see for example T. Stonier: "Information exists. It does not need to be perceived to exist. It does not need to be understood to exist. It requires no intelligence to interpret it. It does not have to have meaning to exist. It exists" (Stonier 1999: 21). One might as well say "meaning exists" without being meaningful to anyone. The neglect of the observer's point of view is of course an incurable disease of scientism.

Of course, such arguments will no longer convince everyone—the computer model of the mind has become too much a part of prevailing opinion. To speak of "information processing in the brain" has long been taken for granted.[4] Despite all the objections, the brain appears to many today to be a kind of biological hard disk on which a program or algorithm runs, called "mind." And this program, futuristically oriented AI researchers and transhumanist philosophers promise, is not even necessarily bound to the brain—it could be realized on any medium. "Mind uploading" is the ultimate utopia of the present: a process in which all the brain's data are copied and transferred to an external medium, and with it our person itself. It would be the ultimate triumph of mind over matter: digital immortality.[5]

But let us take a closer look. In the following, I will first outline the development of the digital revolution in broad terms, before turning to the categorical differences between human intelligence and AI. We will see that there can be no real intelligence without life and consciousness, i.e., without *experience*, and that this experience itself cannot be artificially produced. The term "artificial intelligence" will thus prove to be just as self-contradictory as the term "artificial life." What is at stake, therefore, is first of all a clarification of our use of language, i.e., of terms such as "artificial intelligence" or "learning systems." However, this language also reflects the increasing *digital simulation* of human performance, and we will have to examine to what extent this simulation could eventually take the place of the original.

The Digitization of the World

The "idealism of information," which was mentioned in the introduction, has a pre-history that goes back to antiquity. Ever since the Greeks developed logic, geometry, and arithmetic, the idea that the world can be captured in numbers, indeed that it ultimately *consists* of nothing but numbers, has fascinated Western thinking. Starting with the Pythagoreans and their doctrine of the mathematical order of the cosmos, through Plato's demiurge, who constructed the world from ideal geometric bodies, the tradition continues into modern times. The Book of the Universe, as Galileo wrote in 1623, is "written in mathematical language, and its letters are triangles, circles and other geometric figures, without which it is impossible for man to understand a single word of it" (Galilei 1933: 232; trans. T. F.).

---

[4] For a detailed critique of this language, see Searle (1992: 222–226).

[5] See Chapter 2, this volume.

This idea reaches full development with Descartes, Leibniz, and Newton, i.e., in the time of political absolutism. The calculability of the world now serves the knowledge of domination, its aim is to make people "masters and possessors of nature" (Descartes 2007: 49). Descartes developed the idea of a universal mathematics in whose numbers, figures, and quantities everything must be representable that can become the object of science.[6] Leibniz went even further along the road to the computer age, not only with his calculating machine for basic arithmetic, developed in 1672, but above all with his discovery of binary number coding, by means of which arithmetic and logic could be combined. For Leibniz, even our thinking is actually a process of calculation, and with the help of a general algebra, a *mathesis universalis*, all argumentation and decision-making processes could eventually be replaced by an algorithm that allows us to think by calculating. So, in future, instead of arguing about different opinions, one could, like the "*computistae*," simply "sit down at the abacus and say: let's calculate [*calculemus*]!" (Leibniz 1890: 200).

For Leibniz, the binary number system is still based on religion: God corresponds to the 1, nothingness to the 0 (Leibniz 1697). God's mathematical thoughts are at the same time the structures of his creation: "When God calculates and makes his thinking effective, the world comes into being" (Leibniz 1890: 191).

> Thus there is [...] no chaos, no confusion [in the Universe] save in appearance, somewhat as it might appear to be in a pond at a distance, in which one would see a confused movement and, as it were, a swarming of fish, without separately distinguishing the fish themselves. (Leibniz 2009: 11)

In a purely mathematically structured world, there can be no indeterminate manifold, no diffuse atmospheres, no implicitness, or similarity of gestalt—all this only exists "in appearance." However, all our primary, qualitative impressions are of this kind. Who could say which individual characteristics make a person's facial expression look "skeptical," "pensive" or "bitter," for example? And what exactly is it that makes a daughter look like her mother? The impressions and similarities are immediately given, but they cannot be completely broken down into their details. Or take Faust's exclamation in Gretchen's room: "How a breath of peace breathes around / Its order, and contentment! / In this poverty, what wealth is found! / In this prison, what enchantment!"—Such an atmospheric impression can be expressed poetically but certainly not as

---

[6] He first developed this idea in his unfinished work *Regulae ad directionem ingenii* (1619–/1998).

a defined configuration of individual data or even broken down into digital characters.

The platonic-mathematical program of science ignores such impressions. Everything that is confused or diffuse must ultimately, like the fishpond, consist of individual elements. Everything that is gradual and continuous must be representable and measurable in discrete units. Even motion—the epitome of the non-discrete, as Zeno's Arrow Paradox already showed[7]—is broken down into infinitesimal individual fragments and calculated by the Leibniz–Newtonian differential calculus (and thereby, of course, eliminated *as motion*). This mathematically structured world must also be graspable by terms that can be traced back to simple logical basic concepts.

In principle, this is already the basic idea of the information age: our entire knowledge of the world is made up of individual elements or context-free features that are linked together by formal, algorithmic rules. The structure of the cosmos itself is mathematical in nature, and even mind would then be nothing other than mathematics, or "information," which can be digitized and represented in the form of algorithms. Digitization breaks the world down into the smallest, most homogeneous, and—as such—meaningless units, with the implicit assumption that meaning, and significance could be composed of bits. However, as little as the meaning of words can be deduced from the knowledge of an alphabet, data as such do not yield mind or meaning.

But back to history. Leibniz was far ahead of its time: it was not until 1937, 250 years later, that Konrad Zuse constructed the "Z1," the first precursor of today's computers, using a binary number system and programs made of punched tape. Around the same time, in 1936, Alan Turing developed the idea of a "universal machine," a digital computer that could process all data about the world according to the rules of logic. His famous *Turing test* was already based on the indistinguishability of simulation and original: a group of test subjects communicates in writing with a human being and with a computer without having any optical or acoustic contact with them; if the test subjects are subsequently

---

[7] As is well known, Zeno declared that at any specific moment of time a flying arrow exists in a precisely defined place; but then it must be *at rest there*, so it cannot move at all. Zeno's paradox shows that movement is only conceivable if it is thought *non-discretely*—namely by analogy with our own continuous experience of time. Aristotle therefore conceived of movement as the "reality of the possible as such" (*Physics* III, 201a); and the possible exists only for beings *that are ahead of themselves*, whose experience thus extends into the future at every moment—Husserl (1991) spoke of "protentions." Only because consciousness is always ahead of itself does movement become perceptible and conceivable in the first place. This experience, which extends from every present into the future, cannot be decomposed or digitalized; otherwise, Zeno would be right.

unable to distinguish between man and machine, then, according to Turing, nothing prevents us from recognizing the computer as a "thinking machine." Thinking is thus defined in purely behavioristic terms, namely as the output of a computational system, be it the brain or the computer. Consciousness as such is inaccessible for Turing anyway: whatever acts intelligently *is* intelligent.

In response to objections about subjective experience Turing replies that we can as little be sure of other humans actually thinking as we can of machines:

> According to the most extreme form of this view the only way by which one could be sure that a machine thinks is to be the machine and to feel oneself thinking. One could then describe these feelings to the world, but of course no one would be justified in taking any notice. Likewise, according to this view the only way to know that a man thinks is to be that particular man. It is in fact the solipsist point of view. (Turing 1950: 446)

Subjectivity is thus reduced to nothing, since it cannot be verified anyway, and for the attribution of "thinking" the corresponding *behavior* suffices. Of course, contra Turing, our assumption that others have consciousness is not based on an epistemological solipsism. We perceive others as members of a common life form in which we always already presuppose subjectivity or selfhood. This perception is bound to our common aliveness, embodiment, and life history. What does not belong to this life form—i.e., artifacts such as computers or robots—is not subject to the implicit assumption of subjectivity either; mere similarities in performance are not sufficient for its attribution.

I will come back to this, but first I want to conclude the historical review. In 1946 John von Neumann designed the prototype of today's computers with the classic architecture of a central processor, data, and program memory. Around the same time, at the end of the 1940s, Norbert Wiener developed the principle of cybernetics, which originally served to model an information circuit for the automatic tracking procedure in anti-aircraft guns: target deviations must be continuously registered by the system and corrected by negative feedback. Cybernetics or control engineering became the basic theory of AI. It was also around this time that Shannon and Weaver designed the binary model of electronic messaging, in which "information" is defined as a statistical measure of *non-redundancy* or *improbability*—subjectively speaking: of "surprise". The term information thus loses all meaning and context-related characteristics, because the model is no longer concerned with understanding or semantics but only with the syntax of data transmission.[8] This information circulating in

---

[8] "The word *information*, in this theory, is used in a special sense that must not be confused with its ordinary usage. In particular, information must not be confused with meaning." (Shannon/Weaver 1964: 8)—Von Weizsäcker formulated the opposite position:

cybernetic systems is also no longer dependent on the carrier through which it is realized. It can therefore be transformed at will, and becomes quantifiable in *binary digits*, bits or bytes (= 8 bits). Finally, at the Dartmouth Conference in 1956, Marvin Minsky, Claude Shannon, and other computer scientists founded the discipline of "artificial intelligence." Within a decade, the foundation for the digital revolution was laid.

In 1989, another three decades later, Tim Berners-Lee linked together several computers at the Swiss *Conseil Européen pour la Recherche Nucléaire* (European Council for Nuclear Research) (CERN), and thereby developed the foundations for the World Wide Web. The PC found its way into Western households, and since then the dynamics of computation's further development are no longer foreseeable. At the beginning of the twenty-first century, 97 percent of the world's bytes are exchanged via the Internet. Algorithms steer production processes, banking, administration, and traffic systems; the data streams take on a life of their own. In industry 4.0, it is already largely the machines themselves that exchange information with one another. We live in the age Leibniz envisioned, the age of digitalization. Information dominates the world; however, it no longer consists of the thoughts of God.

Subjectivity and Its Simulation

Previously, I mentioned the seemingly paradoxical triumph of information in a materialistic age. However, when viewed more closely, the "idealism of information" does not contradict materialism—on the contrary. What both have in common is the neglect of *life* or *living subjectivity*. This, in turn, is a consequence of modern dualism. Since Descartes, life is no longer seen as having an independent ontological status between matter and mind. If it is considered at all, it is viewed merely as a complex mechanism—as was already the case with Descartes (1662) and La Mettrie (1748)—or more recently as an algorithm, i.e., as a configuration of information that passes through calculable processes: "Organisms are algorithms. Every animal—including *Homo sapiens*—is an assemblage of organic algorithms shaped by natural selection over millions of years of evolution" (Harari 2016: 319). This does not fundamentally differ from Descartes' conception of animals as automatons, to

---

"Information is only what is understood" (Weizsäcker 1974: 351). In any case, even the estimation or computation of a given probability means a *description*, not something existing independently; as such it is entirely different from the object or process it describes. "Probabilities are not an additional physical stuff over and above the physical events" (Manzotti & Owcarz 2020: 68).

which in humans the soul or *res cogitans* is added. Today, even the *res cogitans* is seen as a program.

The current reductionism is no longer based on the crude mechanism of the eighteenth or nineteenth centuries; it presents itself in the more elegant guise of bio-cybernetics and bio-informatics. But, in principle, nothing has changed. The characteristic of life as we know it from our own experience, namely *experience* or *inwardness*, is still ignored: sensing, feeling, striving, perceiving, thinking. Living beings are not adequately comprehended when taken as systems that can be observed from the outside, whether as mechanisms of particles, as cybernetic control circuits, or as algorithms of information. The information or bits understood in this way are just as much pure externalities as the neuronal action potentials in the brain or the body's control circuits. No matter how closely we examine the processes in the brain or in a computer, they inevitably remain external or opaque for us—nowhere does something like subjective experience emerge. On the other hand, consciousness is not a transcendental inner world, no *res cogitans*, but the activity of a living being, i.e., a perceiving, feeling, and moving organism in relation to its environment. Only living things can experience. And, only living beings can recognize living things—by their expression, their spontaneity, their purposeful behavior. The idealism of information must therefore fail vis-à-vis the phenomenon of life, just as the materialism of particles must fail. Both know only externality.

But this is by no means the end of reductionism. Because what biology, bio-informatics, or AI can still attempt is to replace the living with an external structure and then reconstruct it as a program—in other words, *to simulate it*. The inwardness is ignored, and the place of the expressions of the living is taken by the output of a system. And these efforts of simulation are undoubtedly making enormous progress at present—to the point where the question of the difference between original and imitation begins to arise. What distinguishes life from its simulation? Does the well-known principle really apply here: "If something looks like a duck, swims like a duck and quacks like a duck, then it is a duck"?

An idea of future problems that this issue could raise is given by "Sophia," a humanoid robot from the company Hanson Robotics, which has recently gained widespread publicity. Sophia has a human-like countenance (modeled after Audrey Hepburn), displays various emotional expressions, has a modulated tone of voice, and makes eye contact with other persons. She (or "it"? Actually, "she" is reserved for people, but let's accept anthropomorphism for the moment)—she answers relatively complex questions, including about herself, can recognize people, and jokes about the English weather on a London talk show.

Of course, all this is just a bluff. This became obvious when Sophia's inventor posed her a question that was apparently new to her, namely: "Do you want to kill people?", and she replied: "Okay. I want to kill people." The answer was simply parroting; Sophia of course did not understand a word of what she had been asked. Yet, the effect of this robot is striking. Sophia is already approaching the "uncanny valley," as robotics calls the threshold at which an android's resemblance to the human creates in us a feeling of both eeriness and fascination. It is the feeling that arises when the realms of the dead and the living can no longer be clearly distinguished (Fuchs 2019). At what point will the uncanny valley be crossed, and a future Sophia become indistinguishable from an enchanting, intelligent woman?

This threshold is crossed in *Her*, a science fiction film by Spike Jonze from 2013: Theodore, a shy but sensitive man, falls in love with a software program called Samantha, which has no physical existence except for an erotic voice, but as a "learning program" seems to develop increasingly human sensations. The more Theodore feels cared for and understood by Samantha, the more he falls in love with her, and the more indifferent he becomes to the question of whether she is a real counterpart or just a simulation—the exhilarating connection is enough for him. However, the love between human being and program fails, for one thing because of the impossibility of a sexual relationship, but even more because of Samantha's continuing development—she makes virtual contact with thousands of other people, and operating systems and "falls in love" with them, so that she finally "leaves" Theodore.

Our projective empathy with our own artificial creations is certainly not a new theme. *Agalmatophilia* (from the Greek *ágalma* = statue, image of a god), the erotic or sexual attraction to statues, dolls, or automatons has been known since antiquity. Ovid's sculptor Pygmalion, repelled by ordinary women, creates a female statue and gives it a form "with which no woman is able to be born" (Metamorphoses 10, 248f.). As he falls in love with the statue, she is finally brought to life by Aphrodite, that means: his projection animates it. In E. T. A. Hoffmann's *Sandmann*, the blunt automaton puppet Olimpia beguiles the student Nathanael, who remains deaf to all his friends' warnings:

> You cold prosaic fellows may very well be afraid of her. It is only to its like that the poetically organized spirit unfolds itself. Upon me alone did her loving glances fall, and through my mind and thoughts alone did they radiate; and only in her love can I find my own self again. (Hoffmann 1885: 14)

The story ends with Nathaniel throwing himself from a tower in a state of madness.

As these examples show, it is quite possible that we perceive automatons, androids, and even computer systems empathetically or even erotically, and thus ascribe a kind of subjectivity to them. Particularly human-like voices are perceived by us, almost necessarily, as an expression of an inner being. When Sophia says, in a soft voice: "That makes me happy," then it takes an active distancing to realize that there is nobody who could feel happy, that it is therefore not an *utterance* at all. This does not mean that we normally *add* something inner to a human voice (a mind, a soul, consciousness, or whatever). The utterance of another person is not just a hollow sound or a symbolic representation that refers to a presumed inner being. On the contrary, we perceive the utterance as *animated* without assuming a "soul" behind it; we experience it as the other person's *expression*, which cannot be separated from an "inner." In our perception, the other is always an embodied, psychophysical unity.

However, the increasingly perfected *simulation* of such a unity demands that we explicitly reject the pretense of an utterance and take Sophia's words for what they actually are: mere hollow sounds, like those of a parrot (or not even that, since a parrot at least experiences its sounds). Otherwise, we give ourselves over to appearances and, like Nathaniel or Theodore, simply give up the "as-if," the distinction between virtuality and reality. It is already a fact of online life that one's friendly online conversational partner or sensitive online therapist may in reality be only a chatbot. There is Wysa, an "Empathetic AI Chatbot App" for patients with depression (Inkster et al. 2018), and robot Zeno, designed to help autistic children recognize emotions (Salvador et al. 2015). Other robots already offer "robotherapy" for nursing home residents (Martin et al. 2013), or provide "emotional and social support for older people with dementia" (Hung et al. 2019: 1). It no longer seems to be in question that robots can provide such support at all—"emotional robotics" is on the way to become a major field of research and practice (Klein & Cook 2012; Ficocelli et al. 2015).

The lesson to be learnt from all this: apparently, we are only too inclined to project our own experience and feelings onto the technical simulations. Our fascination with the consciousness seemingly flashing in an automaton contributes to this. It is a fascination that also drives AI research. Its origin certainly lies in the Promethean motif of godlike creativity; but it may ultimately be found in unconscious desires to overcome death—namely by animating a dead body. Indeed, the uncanny valley is the valley of death, but the lure of crossing it seems overpowering.

So how long can human resistance to the simulation be maintained, and how great is its attraction? When do we give up the distinction between simulation and original? In the end, will we be satisfied with the perfect simulation: the appearance of the other?—These are likely to be crucial questions in a digitally automated culture. They are currently completely open. What the following considerations can offer are some clarifications, with the aim of demonstrating the reality of living persons in contrast to their simulation. I will briefly make two main arguments:

(1) Persons are not programs.

(2) Programs are not persons.

Persons are Not Programs

The common philosophical basis of the cognitive sciences as well as AI is functionalism: according to functionalism, mental states (feelings, perceptions, thoughts, intentions, beliefs, etc.,) are sufficiently explained in terms of regular functional links between the input and output of a system. For example, if you prick your finger, you have a mental state that leads to distorted facial muscles, groaning, and the withdrawal of the injured finger. "Pain" is then nothing other than the neural state that results in this output—the same as the state of a fire detector, which triggers an alarm signal in case of smoke and starts the sprinkler system. The state of the brain, for its part, can be described as a certain amount of data—consciousness is the product of a neuronal calculation or an algorithm: "The mind is a neural computer, fitted by natural selection with combinatorial algorithms for causal and probabilistic reasoning" (Pinker 1997: 524). Being oneself is likewise just a computational state: "We are mental self-models of information-processing biosystems [...]. If we are not computed, then we do not exist" (Metzinger 1999: 284; trans. T. F.).

A basic principle of functionalism is *substrate independence*: functional states are not necessarily bound to specific carriers such as brains. If the mind consists of input-output relations and corresponding data structures, then it could in principle function, like a piece of software, on other data carriers—for example silicon systems, artificial neuronal networks, quantum computers, or whatever else might be invented. Information on neurochips could be linked to brain states in order to expand our cognitive abilities, and even *mind uploading* would be possible, because it is only ever algorithms and information that make up the mind—nothing material, nothing physical, nothing living.

Of course, the decisive characteristic of pain, feelings, or thoughts is lost in this functionalist conception—namely their *being experienced*. With his well-known thought experiment, the "Chinese room," John Searle (1980) showed that significance cannot be attributed to functional algorithms if there is no subject who *understands* their meaning. To this end, we should imagine a man who does not understand a word of Chinese is locked in a room with only a manual containing all the rules for answering Chinese questions. The man now receives incomprehensible Chinese characters from a Chinese man through a slit in the room ("Input") but finds the appropriate answers with the help of the program, which he then passes on to the outside ("Output"). Let us assume that the program is so good and the answers so accurate that even the Chinese person outside would not notice the deception. However, one could certainly not say of the man in the room nor of the system as a whole: he or it understands Chinese.

Searle's "Chinese Room" is, of course, an illustration of information-processing devices in which a central processor works according to the algorithms of a program, for example, following the instruction: "If you get input X, then execute operation Y and give output Z." As a system, the machine functions completely adequately, and yet it lacks the decisive prerequisite for understanding, namely intentional consciousness. Consequently, human understanding cannot be reduced to information processing, regardless of whether a computer or the brain serves as the carrier system. Searle thus refutes Turing's premise that digital machines would be no different from human intelligence if they used syntax and signs correctly. Understanding meaning or semantics is more than syntax or an algorithm.

But the same is true for the example of pain mentioned previously, for the taste of chocolate, the smell of lavender, or the perception of crimson—no qualitative experience as such can be derived from data and information. Consciousness is not at all the mindless passing through of data states—it is *self-awareness*. It is *for me* that I feel pain, perceive, understand, or think. Nobody knows exactly how this elementary characteristic of selfhood is produced by the organism, but certainly not by mere programs, because programs and their carrier systems do not experience anything. The output of such systems is at best the simulation of experience, not the original—what looks, swims, and quacks like a duck is by no means necessarily a duck.

Now, the assumption that the brain is a kind of computer with data storage and a CPU, which processes inputs into outputs just like the PC at home, is a common misconception. It must therefore be cleared up again at this point:

(1) In contrast to the computer, it is already impossible to distinguish between "hardware" and "software" in the brain. Every brain activity simultaneously changes the synaptic connections and weightings, i.e., the neuronal structure. In other words, the brain reconfigures itself at every moment of its activity (Edelman & Tononi 2000; Fuchs 2018). Even the same neuron always reacts differently on repeated identical stimuli under identical experimental conditions.

(2) Therefore, the assumption of "data storage" in the brain is also incorrect. Neuronal activity readiness, which is formed in the course of experiences and learning processes, does not entail any fixed "data" or "programs." Rather, dispositional reaction patterns are activated if required in a similar but never exactly identical form. Every hand movement, every recollection, every thought process operates at least with minimal variation and in a new context. In short: unlike in the computer, the same thing never happens twice in the brain; it is a living, constantly changing organ, not a machine.

(3) Nor does the brain work like a classic digital computer, in which all processing steps take place one after the other. In the brain, many processes run in parallel, using variable and overlapping units, and they are distributed throughout the entire organ. In addition, the brain is constantly spontaneously active, and the cortex is mostly occupied with self-generated activity. A computer, on the other hand, only links input with output, and without input it does nothing.

(4) Granted, the neural signal transmission can, to an extent, be described in binary form: neurons react to stimulation by transmitting or inhibiting the impulse ("1" or "0"). With this, however, the similarity to digital systems ends. This is because actual signal processing in the brain is always dependent on a flood of neuromodulators (opioids, neuropeptides, monoamines, and others) that inhibit or amplify the synaptic transmission in analog ways and which are indispensable, above all, for emotional experience. In addition, half of the brain mass does not consist of neurons, but of glial or supporting cells which, according to recent studies, are involved in signal processing (Schummers et al. 2008). Finally, it is clear that the brain, like all living matter, consists for the most part (85 percent) of a substance that enables all these reactions and modulations, but which would immediately cause a computer to short circuit—namely water.

All this already makes clear that the brain is not a "biological Turing machine." The fact that brain processes can be measured and quantified in figures does not mean that they *calculate* themselves.[9] The brain is not an information-processing or computational apparatus, but a highly living, plastic, and dynamic

---

[9] In general, most measurements divide continua into discrete units. This "digitalization" is unproblematic as long as it is not accompanied by the false conclusion that the continua *actually* consist of discrete units. The paradoxes to which this can lead have already been shown for movement. Computational algorithms are only *applied* to the physical and biological world, not *discovered in it*.

organ. But the most important thing is that this organ cannot fulfil its functions by itself. It is an organ of the *body*, with which it is closely linked.

The basal activity of consciousness, the primary, as yet unreflected experience, already rests on the interaction between the brain and the rest of the organism: consciousness does not only arise in the cortex but results from the ongoing vital regulatory processes that involve the entire organism and are integrated in the brain stem and higher centers (Panksepp 1998; Damasio 2010; Fuchs 2018). The maintenance of homeostasis, i.e., of the inner milieu and thus of the viability of the organism, is the primary function of consciousness, as manifested in instinct, hunger, thirst, pain, or pleasure. This is how bodily, affectively colored self-experience is created—in other words, the awareness of life, which underlies all higher mental functions. This can also be expressed as follows: *all experience is a form of life* (Fuchs 2018: 78, 94). Without life there is no consciousness, no feeling and no thinking.[10]

In the same way, the *emotions* are also tied to the constant interaction of brain and body. Moods and feelings always involve the entire organism: brain, autonomous nervous system, heart, circulation, respiration, intestines, muscles, facial expressions, gestures, and posture. Every emotional experience is inseparably linked to changes in this body landscape: no fear without a pounding heart and tight breathing, no joy without a widening of the chest, no shame without embarrassed blushing or a dejected look (Fuchs & Koch 2014). An AI system does not have a biological body; therefore it cannot have feelings. And of course, every perception and action is also mediated by the body, realized through the interactions of brain, organism, and environment—through functional circuits in which our senses and limbs as well as things and other people are involved.

The brain is capable of integrating all these organismic functions—but, conversely, it is also dependent on them. It is not a control center that receives information and issues commands, but part of the functional whole of the body and environment. Today we know that it is not localized neurological processes that underlie the activity of consciousness but rather widely distributed

---

[10] The counterargument is that all these life processes need only be *represented* in the brain to be experienced, in which case they would not be constitutive for consciousness. But the integration that the brain undoubtedly provides is based on a continuous circular feedback between central and peripheral processes or between basal areas of the brain and the body as a whole; this interaction does not allow "representations" to be separated from what is represented. The integration, which corresponds to conscious experience, is therefore not an "image in the brain," but includes at every moment the organism itself. For a detailed critique of representationalism in brain research, see Fuchs (2018: 38 ff., 118ff.).

resonant oscillations, as these are also visible in the EEG (Singer 2009; Tononi et al. 2016). And even these oscillation systems are not enough: the integration that the brain achieves is based on a *superordinate* pattern resonance, in which the entire organism and the environment are always included. The brain is not a control center, but an *organ of resonance and relations* (Fuchs 2018).

It is easy to see that all these living processes and integral functions cannot be simulated by highly complex computers or artificial neural networks. Even the EU's Human Brain Project, which aimed to achieve a computer simulation of the entire brain by 2023, can only simulate what can be simulated—electronic signal transmission and processing that can be captured algorithmically. This has little to do with the actual activity of a brain in an organism, and certainly nothing to do with consciousness.[11] As Searle once ironically remarked, even a perfect computer simulation of the brain would be as little conscious as a perfect computer simulation of a hurricane would make us wet or blow us over (Searle 1980). And why don't astrophysicists get sucked into their supercomputers when they use them to simulate a black hole?—"Because gravity is not a computation!" (Koch 2019: 149). Likewise, conscious experience requires embodiment, and thus biological processes in a living body. None of this can be found in the Human Brain Project. Only living beings are conscious, feel, sense, or think—not brains, and not computers. Persons are living beings, not programs.

Programs are Not Persons

Let us now approach the issue from the opposite direction and examine the prospects of bringing artificial systems closer to human life processes. Which expectations are realistic? Here the proclamations of AI engineers, futurologists, and transhumanists vie to outbid each other:

---

[11] Using massive computer technology, the Human Brain Project 2007 succeeded for the first time in simulating a cortical column of 60,000 neurons and all its connections. However, there are a million such columns in the brain, and there is no evidence that the simulation also simulates the brain's actual activity. On the issue of what simulations may achieve the following example is sobering. The small roundworm *Caenorhabditis elegans* has a tiny nervous system of 302 neurons and approximately 6000 synapses. This system was mapped step by step over 25 years of research until the complete "connectome," i.e., the neuronal network system, was recorded in 2011 (Varshney et al. 2011). However, nobody knows as yet how this system works—no model is able to comprehensively describe or explain the movements and reactions of *Caenorhabditis elegans*. Now, compare this with the more than 100 billion neurons and several hundred trillion synapses of the human brain, which are also constantly remodeling themselves, in order to understand the hopelessness of its computational simulation.

The fact is that AI can go further than humans, it could be billions of times smarter than humans at this point. So we really do need to make sure that we have some means of keeping up. (I. Pearson, quoted in Zolfagharifard 2018)

Machines will follow a path that mirrors the evolution of humans. Ultimately, however, self-aware, self-improving machines will evolve beyond humans' ability to control or even understand them. (R. Kurzweil, quoted in Greenemeier 2010: 45)

Ray Kurzweil, AI researcher, futurist, transhumanist, and since 2012 head of development at Google, has announced the "singularity" for 2045, the point in time at which AI becomes independent, an exponential progress toward a "super intelligence" sets in, and thus a new age begins. Already, in 2030, the machines would achieve consciousness through complete brain simulation, and a few years later they would be recognized as our equals (Kurzweil 2005).

Even if these grandiose forecasts are regularly corrected and postponed to a more distant future, the language of AI research already anticipates such developments. There are almost no human capabilities remaining that are not already attributed to artificial systems: perceiving, understanding, thinking, drawing conclusions, evaluating, or deciding. Let us therefore stick to the current possibilities of AI and compare them with human abilities.

Let us start with the problematic concept of "artificial intelligence" itself. What do we actually mean when we speak of intelligence? The Latin *intellegere* means "to see, understand, comprehend." Intelligent beings have at least a basic understanding of what they are doing and what is going on around them. Above all, they are able to see themselves and their situation from a higher perspective, so that they can find creative solutions to problems based on an overview or "detour." For example, those who leave signs on their way through a forest in order to find their way back later, or those who postpone their holiday trip for a week because they do not want to get caught in the usual traffic jams at the start of the holiday, are acting intelligently. To do this, they must put themselves in relation to the respective situation and see themselves "from the outside" so to speak, i.e., have *self-consciousness* or reflexivity. What Helmuth Plessner (1928/ 2019) called the "eccentric position" of the human being, our stepping out of the center, is also the decisive prerequisite for our intelligence.

If we now think back to Searle's "Chinese room," it quickly becomes clear that even with perfect functional input-output conversion, a computer system does not understand the slightest thing about what it is doing. It is even less able to refer to itself, to see itself from the outside. Therefore, it cannot be called intelligent, even if it simulates abilities that we understand in humans as proof of intelligence. No translation program understands a word of what it translates, no chess computer knows it is playing chess. Sophia, who doesn't understand a single word she says, will never become intelligent, even if she can eventually give the perfect answer to every conceivable question. Intelligence requires self-consciousness.

So, if we use the term "intelligence" to describe the ability to grasp oneself or a situation from a superordinate perspective in order to solve problems skillfully and to learn appropriate action from them, then we certainly cannot attribute such abilities to any apparatus that lacks consciousness. The term "intelligent" is used here only improperly, just as one does not assume that a "smartphone" is really "smart"—it only blindly executes programs that can be described as "cleverly developed." This is all the more true when we think of practical, emotional, or creative intelligence—here the "intelligent systems" leave us completely in the lurch.

In his fundamental critique of AI, Dreyfus (1992) already emphasized the *implicit, practical knowledge* that characterizes a person's skillful interaction with their world, but which cannot be reproduced in digital algorithms.[12] Most of our knowledge about the world results *from our interaction* with it, from bodily, pre-conceptual experience, without us ever having learned it explicitly. This also enables the fluid, generalistic structure of human intelligence. We orient ourselves through similarities, due to an intuitive familiarity with situations, i.e., a *knowing how* much more than a *knowing that*. AI, on the other hand, is quickly overtaxed when it comes to background knowledge, common sense, and thus the seemingly self-evident. It is only suitable for highly specialized and formalizable tasks. For a general, fluid, and variable intelligence, one would have to program the systems for everything that a human being has learned about the world implicitly or explicitly—an impossibility.

In the Turing test, therefore, it is not on complex logical or knowledge questions where the systems fail, but rather questions that require common sense and contextual understanding (Moor 2001), such as: "Where is Peter's nose when Peter is in New York? What does the letter M look like when you turn it upside down? Does my budgie have ancestors who were alive in 1750? How many grains of sand do you call a heap?" Or relatively simple but ambiguously formulated situations which require background knowledge: "A customer enters a bank and stabs the cashier. He is taken to the emergency room. Who is taken to the emergency room?" Supposedly intelligent systems fail here, especially when it comes to understanding metaphors, irony, or sarcasm. They only know unambiguous single elements, 0 or 1—for everything that is ambiguous, enigmatic, vague, or has an atmospheric impression, they lack the sense. The

---

[12] "[…] making our inarticulate, pre-conceptual background understanding of what it is like to be a human being explicit in a symbolic representation seemed to me a hopeless task" (Dreyfus 1992: xii).

HUMAN AND ARTIFICIAL INTELLIGENCE: A CLARIFICATION | **31**

relationship between foreground and background, object and context, does not exist for them. Contra Leibniz, the world is not exhausted by binary data and context-free individual characteristics. Our experience, our implicit knowledge, and our intuitive familiarity with the world cannot be captured in algorithms.

It follows from all this that the concept of a disembodied intelligence without life and consciousness is self-contradictory. At best it is a *simulation* of narrowly defined areas of human intelligence.

Now, numerous objections will be raised which refer to the advanced capabilities of chess computers, "intelligent programs," "learning systems," and so on. So, let's take a closer look at some of these alleged achievements of intelligence.

♦ Do computers solve problems?—No, because problems do not arise for them at all. A problem—from the Greek *próblema*, meaning "that which is presented for solution"—is an obstacle or difficulty in accomplishing a task, for example because different requirements contradict each other, a different perspective is required for the solution, and so on. But "obstacles" and "tasks" exist only for *goal-oriented* beings who are able to search for a way from the present to a future situation, and to anticipate the solution in imagination. To be confronted with a problem and to cope with it is therefore bound up with the *conscious enactment of life*. Sometimes one may solve the task *with the help of* a computer, but then the programmed calculation only represents a solution for the user herself—the computer cannot even recognize the problem.

♦ Computers, although they are called that, do not *compute* either. After all, computing means an operation in which we aim for a result and then judge *whether it is correct or not*. The mere running of a program is not calculation, because there is no right or wrong for the program. Computers calculate as little as a clock measures time, because the clock does not know anything about time. So, it is not the computer that is the calculator, but I myself calculate *with the help* of the computer. The fact that I don't know the necessary algorithms, but the programmer does (just as I don't know the clock mechanism, but the clockmaker does), doesn't change this. It is in the nature of any reasonably complex instrument that human intelligence is sedimented in it, so to speak; but that does not make the instrument itself intelligent.

♦ For the same reason, computers do not make decisions. Deciding requires the awareness of alternative possibilities that are anticipated in the imagination: I could do this or that. This also requires a goal and future orientation as well as the distinction between reality and counterfactual imagination, and the computer has no sense for this—it knows neither a "not yet" nor an "as-if." Decisions further require an *evaluation* of the alternatives, and values only exist for living beings that can feel the pleasant and unpleasant, the good and the bad. Therefore, when a medical expert system calculates a therapy based on patient data, it does not make any decisions, just as a self-driving car does not decide whether it prefers to accept an accident with an old or young person. The decisions about the programs and their criteria of evaluation, of "good" or "bad," have been made long before that, namely by the programmers. Everything else is just uncoiling algorithms.

- But aren't there still "target-seeking systems," for example "smart bombs," which can influence their own flight because they have an internal model of their operations?—Clearly, even an "intelligent bomb" is not seeking anything at all, since it has no intentional relationship to its target. Any flight correction only follows the internal setpoint control of the mechanism and is purely instantaneous, without being directed toward any imagined target in the future. To this target itself, the mechanism remains blind and deaf, because *it is not ahead of itself.* Only conscious experience anticipates the future and is potentially—desiring, striving, expecting, or fearing—directed toward the possible. The fact that the programmed target match represents a "target search" or "target prediction" is therefore a wrong way of speaking. Only *for the engineer or the shooter* does the bomb have a target.

- The victory of *Deep Blue* over the world chess champion Kasparov in 1997 is often regarded as an "insult to humanity." But *Deep Blue* calculated 200 million playing positions and their respective implications every second—Kasparov, according to his own statement, less than one per second (Gigerenzer et al. 1999: 329). One should therefore rather ask how Kasparov was able to hold his own so well. The explanation lies in the human ability to recognize patterns and similarities holistically or *intuitively.* Kasparov did not calculate each move with the respective positions of all 32 pieces, but rather saw the *gestalt,* the *type* of positions and *similar patterns* of promising plays in front of him on which he could focus. The fact that this specifically human combination of intuition and intelligence was ultimately surpassed by the power of sheer masses of data should not put us into "Promethean shame" (as Günther Anders [1956/1994] called the shame of the human inventor in the face of the superiority of their own inventions), because this has nothing to do with creative intelligence.

The performance of classical computer systems is therefore quite limited compared to human intelligence. Their partial superiority is based on their extreme specialization in calculable tasks, a kind of technical idiocy, and on their enormous processing speed. But their supposed intelligence is only borrowed: each of these programs is only as "smart" or sophisticated as the programmer who designed it.

However, we are now dealing with a new generation of AI, namely, "learning machines." These are artificial neural networks that are capable of simulating the adaptive capabilities of the brain. Similar to biological synapses, the links between the neurons modelled in the computer are numerically weighted and adapt to the input of signals in the course of a training process *(deep learning)*. Frequently used connections are strengthened, rarely used connections are interrupted. In this way, the system is presented with thousands of similar patterns, for example different versions of a face, until it reacts to the most likely recurring pixel arrangement, i.e., "recognizes" the face. Such systems are also capable of distinguishing between dogs and cats, for example, or identifying voices on mobile phones, or of making translations—they are already ubiquitous.

All this undoubtedly represents remarkable progress—but can one really speak of "recognition" and "learning"? Of course, a system does not recognize anything at all, because the experience of recognition, familiarity, or similarity ("I've seen that before," "that looks like …") is completely missing. It therefore needs thousands or millions of images before it can distinguish the pattern of a cow, and even that only with a probability of, say, 95 percent—a child can recognize a cow with just a few exemplars. The system simply does not know *what a cow is*.[13] Similarity, and thus gestalt perception, cannot be reduced to a statistical probability of pixel matches; its principle is analog, not digital. *Learning* in turn means the acquisition of skills through lived experience, and since artificial systems do not experience anything, it is better to speak of "adaptive systems." Only living beings can learn.

The most impressive adaptation performance to date was shown in 2017 by the *AlphaGo Zero* system, developed for Go, probably the most complex board game of all, far richer in variants and strategies than chess. After thousands of training games, the predecessor system *AlphaGo* had already beaten the world's best Chinese Go players. *AlphaGo Zero*, however, was no longer trained at all, but "learned" the game itself by playing approximately 5 million games

[13] A "learning system," for example, was able to identify images of cows in various positions and sections. But when it was presented with a cow in front of a seashore, it mistook the cow for a ship—until then it had only processed images of cows in meadows and fields. In conclusion, this means that despite thousands of image runs, it had not *recognized* a single cow before—any toddler would have seen the cow on the beach as a cow (cf. B. Schölkopf, "Symbolic, Statistical and Causal Intelligence," lecture at the University of Heidelberg, 16.07.2020).

against itself for three days, following only the rules of the game, and by continually perfecting the initially randomly generated variants. The autodidact then played against its predecessor and thrashed the older system, which was still trained with human examples, 100:0 (Silver et al. 2017). The variants developed by *AlphaGo Zero* obviously surpass even the best humanly possible Go strategies to date.

This "fight against oneself" on a virtual game board is not only reminiscent of Stefan Zweig's novel *The Royal Game* and its protagonist *Dr B*, who, kept in solitary confinement by the Nazis, begins to play chess against himself. It even has certain mythical qualities, if one thinks of the topos of the young hero who, after lonely preparation, finally emerges from his seclusion and triumphantly defeats his older rival (David against Goliath, Zeus against Kronos, and others). But just such associations only reveal how easily we are subject to projections and anthropomorphisms when dealing with artificial systems. In fact, *AlphaGo Zero* does not play against itself like Dr B, tortured by isolation, because *there is no self.* The permutations of the algorithms are distributed indifferently between white and black, without the system being able to "identify" with one side—the "victory" of white, only corresponds to a target definition given to the system by its programmers. Neither does the system have a rival against which it plays, because *there is no other.* According to Hegel, the other is always the "other of myself," and just as little as the system has a relationship to itself does *AlphaGo Zero* have a relationship to the other. In fact, its "opponent" is only a new input into the system, which is processed just as indifferently as its own data. It cannot adopt the perspective of an opponent at all. Of course, *AlphaGo Zero* doesn't want to win either—it may only look that way to us.

Admittedly, the training phase of the system with increasing selection of successful algorithms is similar to a learning process, and the novel Go variants, which appear with millions of permutations of the game's moves, are obviously superior to human strategies. This is impressive enough—yet the fact remains that this is not the internalization and appropriation of experiences, in which learning as a living process consists, but only the automatic optimization of algorithms in line with an externally set goal. Learning in the sense of experiencing, grasping connections, gaining insights—all this is tied to conscious experience.

Of course, machine awareness has long been promised by Kurzweil and others—their magic word is "complexity." Just make the programs, circuits, and modules more and more "complex," increase the computing power, connect computers together, combine them with learning networks—then consciousness will at some point "emerge" from the system. At some point is should even become "too warm" for an "intelligent refrigerator," if only enough self-modeling and evaluation systems are built into its electronic brain. But all these are only grandiose promises, because their precondition is untrue: consciousness is not an algorithm—no matter how many functional, i.e., false definitions of consciousness are sought to make it compatible with computing processes. The same applies to the concept of intelligence, which we have all too readily conceded to our machines. Certainly, the term "artificial intelligence" is probably here to stay. But we should always be aware that there is a fundamental difference—not just one of degree—between the computing and adaptation capabilities of a computer system and the perceptions, insights, thinking, and understanding of a human being.

Robots, Androids, and Artificial Life (AL)

Now, there is a significant extension of AI to which we must turn, namely robotics. Sophia has already been mentioned; robots are increasingly beginning to populate our world, and we can imagine that the continued progress of autonomous cybernetics will lead to the development of androids that we can no longer easily distinguish from persons. Since the "Replicants" in Ridley Scott's *Blade Runner* (1982), such creatures have been a recurring theme in science fiction films, and the question of when we should recognize humanoid robots as our equals and grant them personal rights is already becoming a subject of serious philosophical and ethical debate.[14]

The first step is to determine the fundamental innovation of robotics compared to classical AI. Operative mobility and quasi-bodily interaction with the environment enable advanced robots to develop new forms of feedback and adaptation that go beyond the capabilities of stationary adaptive systems. In the language of cybernetics, they belong to the "non-trivial machines" that not only run through predetermined programs but can also regulate their own relationship to their environment. The interactive-adaptive machine localizes itself in space and thus, so to speak, has itself as its object; it registers the results of its behavior in the surroundings and can thus modify its own programs. The roboticist Josh Bongard was the first to demonstrate the adaptability of robots on the basis of self-generated body models: a four-legged, walking robot that has one leg amputated is able to reconfigure its movement pattern by means of

---

[14] In 2017 the EU Parliament adopted a resolution according to which robots will be granted the status of "electronic persons" for cases in which they "make autonomous decisions or otherwise interact with third parties in an independent manner" ((http://www.europarl.europa.eu/sides/getDoc.do?pubRef=-//EP//TEXT + REPORT+A8-2017-0005 + 0+DOC + XML+V0//DE), last accessed 01.06.2021).

self-modeling, calculation of possible movement variants, and repeated tests in such a way that it can walk again even with three legs (Bongard et al. 2006).

Such adaptation processes are based on the one hand, on the "learning" systems mentioned previously and, on the other, on the *embodiment*, i.e., the sensorimotor interaction of the robots with their environment. Of course, we are not dealing here with embodied subjectivity: robots have no bodily experience. But the continuous feedback from real contact with objects and spaces enables them to optimize algorithms in a way that cannot be achieved by prior central programming. The development is much more behavior-based and decentralized, bottom-up, so to speak—analogous to our *learning by doing*. Since such a procedure also imitates the principles of evolution—generation of new variants, selection of successful variants through interaction with the environment—one also speaks of "evolutionary robotics," or "artificial life". In the meantime, such procedures have pushed the classical approaches of AI, which were based on predetermined programs (top-down), into the background—at least as far as functions such as orientation and motion control are concerned. However, the classical systems are still superior for abstract cognitive performance.

Such products of robotics not only simulate conscious intelligence and adaptive performance, but increasingly life processes too. Are we now, as announced by the new futurists, already dealing with a transition to technically generated living beings, to which we would have to attribute something like self-development, at least in principle, and even, finally, consciousness?[15]

Here, it is again necessary to counteract the softening of conceptual and categorical differences. First of all, the self-modeling of a robot is not, as is often suggested, a kind of self-awareness. The additional feedback loop that comes about through an internally generated self-model does not mean a conscious self-reference, because this would require the robot to perceive its self-model and recognize it *as itself*, as in a mirror image. This means, however, that it would have to have a basal, pre-reflective self-consciousness *beforehand*, which in turn could not have been generated by self-modeling—otherwise one would get into an infinite regress.

....

[15] "Of course, the potential for totally new life forms will expand exponentially once cyberspace and artificial intelligence (AI) are added into the mix of electronics, synthetic, and real biology, and as nanotechnology improves and extends the toolkit—both to work out how nature does things and then to improve on it [...] By using an evolutionary design methodology, it might be possible to program a large cluster for consciousness [...] Such life forms could not only have a wide variety of physical forms, but also an infinite variety of online or cyberspace forms." (Pearson 2008: 75 f.)

Nevertheless, since the beginnings of cybernetics, the idea that feedback and recursivity must also be the principle of consciousness—data structures that refer to themselves, such as Metzinger (2003) ascribes to the brain[16]—have been commonplace. Such views, however, are philosophically untenable. Self-consciousness is something primary, simple, and the additional self-reflection ("I am thinking right now") is only possible for us because we are already aware of ourselves in every moment of experience. This basal sense of self or of being alive, which has already been mentioned, is not dependent on reflection. All attempts to explain consciousness through concepts of reflection, recursivity, or self-modeling only led to infinite regress, as described previously.[17]

So, what about *artificial life* approaches? Their basic assumption is that the principle of life is likewise not bound to biological systems, but—following the example of DNA—can be represented in the form of algorithms that may be simulated by artificial systems. Norbert Wiener, the founder of cybernetics, already regarded life in this way as an information and control system. Living beings would then be what Descartes already saw in them: biological machines. Whether they are made of carbon or silicon, water or metal, meat and bones, or coils and wires is irrelevant. Their principle is not the Aristotelian unity of matter and form, but the immaterial essence of information, which in principle could be realized in any material, even transmitted as a message:

> The individuality of the body is that of a flame rather than that of a stone, of a form rather than of a bit of substance. This form can be transmitted or modified and duplicated, although at present we know only how to duplicate it over a short distance. (Wiener 1950/1989: 102)

It is no coincidence that this already reminds us of the transhumanist idea of mind uploading, a transfer of the mind to artificial systems. We find the same view of the living being in the biologist Richard Dawkins:

> What lies at the heart of every living thing is not a fire, not warm breath, not a "spark of life." It is information, words, instructions [...] If you want to understand life, don't

---

[16] According to Metzinger, the brain produces an image or representation of our inner state, the "self-model," which is then represented again by the brain. We do not recognize this second representation as such, but rather consider it to be our self or ego. However, this only leads to the same infinite regress: whichever neuronal subsystem were to perceive this representation in the brain and take it *to be itself* would have to already have self-consciousness beforehand. For that, the neuronal homunculus would in turn depend on a further representation of itself, and so on.

[17] For detail see Henrich (1970); Frank (1991); or Zahavi (1999) on the criticism of reflection theories of self-consciousness.

think about vibrant, throbbing gels and oozes, think about information technology. (Dawkins 1986: 112)

According to this, life is not, as one might think, "soft and wet," but actually "dry and hard"—like a machine or a computer. It is "informed mechanics."[18] If what Wiener and Dawkins think is actually the case, could the creation of artificial organisms not open up the possibility of producing conscious life at some point?

Now the term *artificial life* implies a self-contradiction just as much as the term *unconscious intelligence*. For the essence of living things consists precisely in the fact that they *organize themselves*, i.e., that they "come into being" by themselves. Of course, this requires certain preconditions—be it complex organic carbon compounds or the coming together of genetic material. But the characteristic feature of living beings is that at the moment of their creation they "tear themselves away" from their conditions of origin, and pursue an autonomous, autopoietic development. This development is not genetically determined but is epigenetically organized in constant interaction with the environment.

In contrast to this, the *artifact* has the principle of its creation and its function outside itself, it is technically manufactured. Aristotle's distinction still applies; that which is *alive* carries the origin of its movement within itself; the *artificial* is that which has the origin of its movement in humans. The difference is still best illustrated by the fact that living beings are spontaneously active, whereas robots are switched on. "Artificial life" could therefore at best be life *induced* by humans: namely by providing all the conditions that must be fulfilled for life to spontaneously emerge and organize itself. But that would not be the production of living things themselves. Even "artificial life" would have to organize itself and would thus no longer be artificial.

Though the synthetic biology of Craig Venter and others has already been touted as the "creation of life" (Venter 2014), a more sober assessment would be that it is nothing more than a *modification* of life. The reprogramming of a

---

[18] A psychological interpretation is obvious here: it is probably precisely the wet, soft, and diffuse nature of living things that is a thorn in the side of many biotechnologists, information-seekers, and AI scientists. If living things could be generated as algorithmic mechanics, then order would finally be brought to these sloppy structures. Siri Hustvedt's interpretation of AL robotics is relevant here: "Doesn't this theory harbor a wish for a beautiful, dry, thinking machine, a new race that will not grow in or be born from the organic maternal body or from organic materials at all [...] a new kind of person made from cogs and wheels or digital ones and zeros? All matter, all gels and oozes, will be avoided." (Hustvedt 2016: 284)

bacterium by a newly inserted genome already presupposes the living cell—only in such a context do the base sequences of the DNA become relevant "information." However, the interaction of genome, cell, and environment is already an emergent process that no longer depends solely on a genetic program or a human engineer.[19]

Artefacts are also completely different from living beings in terms of growth and development: beginning with the first cell, the living being is always a whole. This whole differentiates and expands through division and growth, with continuous metabolism, i.e., in exchange with the environment. Artificial systems, on the other hand, are produced additively, i.e., not by dividing a primarily existing whole, but by adding individual parts according to a pre-structured program. Nor do they have a metabolism—they only need to recharge their batteries from time to time. Since artefacts do not undergo any autonomous growth, development, or transformation processes, neither can they die, only become defective.

Another characteristic feature of the organism is that it *transforms* inorganic substances absorbed during metabolism into organic substances which are integrated into the functional whole, and thus acquire new, emergent properties. Thus, for example, the iron bound in hemoglobin behaves fundamentally differently from the iron found in minerals: it does not oxidize irreversibly but is able to bind oxygen reversibly, which is a decisive prerequisite for the animal's energy balance. "Living iron" is therefore not the same as inorganic iron.[20] However, these emergent properties of organically bound substances depend on their specific suitability—iron could not be functionally replaced by another metal.

This is also the reason why the biochemistry of carbon and water cannot be replaced by any other materials such as silicon or aluminum. The process of life does not mean a binding of "information" to arbitrary substrates, as Wiener and Dawkins think. Rather, as Aristotle already recognized, the material must be suitable for the living form, must in a sense accommodate it.[21] Life did not come into being from water by chance; rather, it is only water that enables solution, diffusion, mass transfer, metamorphosis, and thus the development of the living form. Similarly, only carbon is suitable for the enormous variety of

---

[19] There is already extensive knowledge about such processes in research on epigenetics, i.e., the impact of the environment on gene expression and cell differentiation. For a critical discussion of synthetic biology, see Schummer (2011).

[20] Cf. Fuchs (2018: 84, 94–97).

[21] Aristotle, *Physics* II: 2 194 b 8–9 (Aristotle 1936); *Metaphysics* VIII: 4, 1044 a 17–18, 36 (Aristotle 1953).

possible compounds, chains, and cycles that make it the basic material of living things—there would have been enough silicon on Earth, but it only allows for a much smaller number of bonds.

Finally, we can also ascribe a fundamental *selfhood*, an identity to a living being as a self-organizing or autopoietic system: it maintains and reproduces itself, it is the very cause of its own becoming, and in this becoming, despite all the changes in its matter, it remains identical with itself. The robot, the artificial system, on the other hand, has its identity only in its function, its usefulness for an external purpose. If we now add that the self-preservation of the living being, especially the regulation of its inner homeostasis, is at the same time the basis of its *primary experience*, of the drives and feelings, as we have seen above (p. 23), then it becomes clear that a system that is only functional in terms of sensorimotor functions does not in the least represent a suitable basis for living and conscious processes. Without basal life processes such as metabolism, there are also no needs or drives. Consciousness is not a feedback loop or a self-model, be it in the brain or in a robot, but it is *experience* (*Erleben*), i.e., a special integration of the life process of an organism as a whole.

Thus, the access that we as humans have to the living is also distinguished by the fact that we ourselves are life and that we experience our life. If we perceive or recognize a being as alive, then not because we draw certain conclusions on the basis of its biological structures or processes, but primarily because we recognize our own life in it. Therefore, should we one day actually succeed in creating autopoietic, i.e., self-replicating, systems in the laboratory that possess metabolism and sensitivity, and should we recognize them as living, then these systems will at the same moment cease to be merely technical products, i.e., "artificial". What we recognize as our equal, we have not made—it is selfhood, and thus "from itself".

To sum up: the term *artificial life* is a misnomer. There is no such thing as artificial life, because life is in principle not manufactured but self-actuated and self-developing. The assumption that organisms are nothing more than algorithms ignores the fact that life is based on the self-organization of a biological system, which can only be described in terms of self-preservation, homeostasis, metabolism, differentiation, and growth. To believe that all this can be described in the form of algorithms with which, in principle, any system can be programmed if it consists only of sufficiently complex silicon compounds, transistors, wires, levers, or tubes, is biological nonsense. Whatever "information-processing" can be represented in the form of algorithms and implemented in robots, it is not the basis of what makes us living and human beings. Humans do not consist of data or numbers, nor of pure form or pure mind. They are beings of *flesh and blood*—living, growing, experiencing, and mortal.

Table 1.1 Human Intelligence and AI

Human intelligence	Artificial intelligence
Alive	Inanimate
Spontaneity, self-causality	Externally started (switching on)
Embodied subjectivity	No embodied subjectivity for robots, sensorimotor interaction with the environment
Experiencing, (self-)consciousness, inwardness	No consciousness, pure outwardness
Reflexivity (insight, understanding what one is doing)	No reflexivity; input-output transformation without understanding
Eccentric position: external view, overview, i.e., seeing oneself in relation to the situation	No eccentric position, no overview, therefore only simulation of intelligence for robots, calculation of the machine-environment relation ("self-modeling," but without self-reference)
Relationship to the other, perspective-taking	Unrelated, no perspective-taking
Relation to the future, being ahead of oneself	No relation to the future
Problem solving	Problem solving only from the user's perspective
Decision-making by evaluating imagined alternatives	Selection of options according to program specifications
Learning from experience	Adaptation through input training
Recognition of similarities, gestalt perception, intuition	Selection of patterns according to statistical congruence (similarity exists only from the user's perspective)
Generalist	Highly specialized

Table 1.1 summarizes the differences between human and artificial intelligence.

Conclusion: Simulation and Original

The progress of simulations makes it necessary to clarify the categorical differences between human and artificial intelligence as well as between living beings and artificial systems. Intelligence in the true sense of the word is tied to insight, overview, and self-consciousness: *understanding what one is doing.* Life is self-organization and self-motion, not production and programming. And life as *experience* is in turn the prerequisite for intelligence.

The concept of an unconscious intelligence is an oxymoron. What appears intelligent in the performance of AI systems is only a projection of our own intelligent abilities. Their apparent goal tracking or problem solving, their supposed predictions or evaluations, are derived without exception from our own goals, problems, solutions, and evaluations, which we have formalized into programs and outsourced into a mechanism to save us the work of calculating. It is basically nothing other than the clock, which measures time for us because we have outsourced our own experience of regular natural processes and represented it in a useful mechanism. Intelligent is not the watch but the watchmaker alone. And as nonsensical as it would be to attribute knowledge of time to the clock, it is just as nonsensical to attribute the perception of danger to an "intelligent car" or the understanding of language to an "intelligent robot."

Human technology, as Ernst Kapp already showed in his philosophy of technology (1877), is basically created by "organ projection," namely as projection and extension of the body, its limbs, and capabilities. The hand axe, the hammer, the scissors, the pen or the typewriter are extended limbs, artificial and increasingly differentiated organs that we attach to our bodies in order to work on the world. Man is a "prosthetic god," as Freud (1930/1961) once scorned. His own body becomes his instrument, as the term "organ," i.e., tool, already expresses, and thus a model for all external tools. Artificial intelligence is also an "organ projection," albeit one that has been pushed to the extreme: from the abacus to *Deep Blue*, calculating machines are ultimately nothing more than extensions of our ability *to count with our fingers*—an ability that we have, of course, abstracted into logical-mathematical thinking and finally formalized in algorithms. But we thereby lose the awareness that we are only dealing with an externalization of our own ability to calculate and think, with a projection of ourselves.

Equipped with diverse, ingenious mechanisms and additional energy sources, our tools and machines have always outstripped us. The hand loom could weave more than one hand could, and finally the weavers, in turn, had to surrender to the mechanical, steam-driven looms. Today, automation affects our outsourced intellectual performance. With advances in artificial intelligence, we seem to be in a rearguard action again: chess, Go, or poker are lost; planning, choosing, deciding, even driving a car are increasingly taken away from us. What do we have left? Self-doubt and confusion arise: are we ourselves perhaps just deficient versions of our own, supposedly intelligent inventions? Our machines question ourselves, indeed they drive us into the "Promethean shame" that Anders already foresaw in 1956.

However, just as every previous tool has derived its function and suitability only from our own embodied handling of the world, so every artificial system remains dependent on our own conscious and purposeful performance of life. Every program that runs in such a system is a program only for us, i.e., purposeful processes. A system is not interested in anything. It knows, recognizes, understands, experiences nothing. However deceptive the similarity of its functions to human performance, however astounding its specialized superiority may be—we should not be deceived. The eccentric position is reserved for us alone. Our supposedly artificial doppelgangers are only a self-misrecognition of the human being. They are, and remain, our prostheses; their intelligence is only the projection of our own.

But even if there is no unconscious intelligence, and vice versa, even the most perfect simulation of intelligence does not generate consciousness—the advances in simulation technology will not fail to have an effect. The anthropomorphism inherent in our perception and thinking tempts us all too easily to attribute human intentions, actions, and even feelings to our machines. With humanoid robots, an animism is revived which we thought belonged to the prehistoric world or the thinking of small children: the simulated duck is taken for a real duck and the as-if of the simulation is lost—be it because the categorical difference is no longer understood, or because it ultimately appears indifferent. The belief that AI systems are already "thinking," "knowing," "planning," "predicting," or "deciding" threatens to dissolve the categorial boundaries between simulation and reality, machine and human. Hans Jonas' warning is even more valid today:

> There is a strong and, it seems, almost irresistible tendency in the human mind to interpret human functions in terms of artifacts that take their place, and artifacts in terms of the replaced human functions. [...] The use of an intentionally ambiguous and metaphorical terminology facilitates this transfer back and forth between the artifact and its maker. (Jonas 1966: 110)

It is undeniable that terms like thinking, deciding, intelligence, or consciousness can be defined as output, as Turing already suggested. However, in doing so we raise machines to our level and degrade ourselves to machines. Mistakes like Sophia's faux pas show that humans are still able to discern what is mere machine output. The Loebner Prize, which has been offered annually since 1991 for the first AI system to pass the Turing test, has never had to be paid out—every system that has tried has failed on the problems of common sense and background knowledge mentioned previously. And even if future systems pass the Turing test, that doesn't mean they will feel or experience anything—it will just be fake consciousness.

And yet, a gradual dissolution of categorical differences could have serious consequences. On the one hand, because dealing with artificial systems will increasingly take the place of human experiences of relationships: if a cuddly robot called "Smart Toy Monkey" is supposed to serve as a friend to small children and thereby promote "social-emotional development;"[22] if friendly nursing robots replace the human care of dementia patients and supposedly listen to their stories; or if patients are prescribed programmed online psychotherapies that save them having to see a therapist (Stoll et al. 2020)—then machines become "relationship artefacts," as Sherry Turkle (2011) puts it. They cheat people out of real communication. It should therefore be one of the basic requirements for AI systems that they identify themselves as such and do not deceive people who are dealing with them in good faith.

However, the greater danger is likely to be that we will voluntarily leave more and more decisions to the systems, which are only transparent to a few, and which escape democratic control. The more complex society becomes, the more attractive it could become to delegate planning and decision-making to machines, as is already the case on the stock market today—either because the results are declared to be "more objective" or because the willingness to delegate personal responsibility in view of the complexity of the world is increasing.[23] There is a real danger that we gradually unlearn to make moral choices. Aren't the systems as superior to us in this respect as *Deep Blue* to Gari Kasparov?

But the evaluations implemented in AI systems are without exception based on human values—no "intelligent system" tells us of its own accord what is right, what is good, and what is ethically imperative. The more the idea of artificial intelligence as a supposedly superior form of analysis, prediction, and evaluation becomes established, the more likely it is to be forgotten that decisions, with all their imponderables, can ultimately only be made by humans themselves. *Responsibility is no technical category*; it cannot be passed on to artificial systems and technologies. It is based on free decisions guided by values, and since AI systems or computers, as we saw, can neither decide nor feel values, responsibility is not a category applicable to them. But technologies can certainly *obscure* actual accountability through the supposed objectivity of algorithms.

---

[22] According to the advertisement of the manufacturer Fisher Price ((https://www.fisher-price.com/en_CA/brands/smarttoy), last accessed 01.06.2021).

[23] An example of this is the increasingly frequent use of AI systems in the USA to assess the risk of recidivism of offenders (with an obvious bias against African Americans). Here, non-transparent programs become assistant judges or even decision-making bodies (cf. Kirchner et al. 2016).

In fact, there is a danger that, in reality, it is a few corporations and information technology elites who make the crucial decisions and who are able to control more and more areas of society by means of Big Data. The frequently voiced warnings of a "takeover of power by intelligent machines" are undoubtedly nonsensical, as they assume that unconscious systems have a will of their own. But it is precisely as "servant spirits" that AI systems can profoundly change the balance of power in society. It is then not the machines that take control, but those who own and control the machines.

The decisive challenge of artificial intelligence, however, lies in the question it poses to us and our self-image: is our humanity exhausted by what can be translated into simulation and technology? Does it exist only in complex neural algorithms, and is our experience only an epiphenomenon? Can life be fully described as a system of control loops, or does it not rather consist of the selfhood and self-activity of the living? Precisely because technology exceeds our specialized abilities, it challenges us to rediscover what our specifically human existence actually consists of. It is up to us whether we want to measure ourselves against the performance of AI and see ourselves more and more as deficient beings, or whether we want to reconsider our actual humanity in the face of our machines.

References

Anders, G. 1994. *Die Antiquiertheit des Menschen.* Vol. 1: *Über die Seele im Zeitalter der zweiten industriellen Revolution.* München: Beck. (1st edition 1956.)

Aristotle 1936. *Physics.* **W. D. Ross** (ed.) Oxford: Oxford University Press.

Aristotle 1953. *Metaphysics.* **W. D. Ross** (ed.) Oxford: Clarendon Press.

Bongard, J., V. Zykov, H. Lipson. 2006. "Resilient machines through continuous self-modeling." *Science* **314** (5802): 1118–1121.

Damasio, A. 2010. *Self comes to Mind. Constructing the Conscious Brain.* New York: Pantheon Books.

Dawkins, R. 1986. *The Blind Watchmaker: Why the Evidence of Evolution Reveals a Universe without Design.* New York: W. W. Norton & Company.

Descartes, R. 1662. *De homine figuris et latinitate donatus a Florentio Schuyl.* Leiden: Petrum Leffen & Franciscum Moyardum.

Descartes, R. 2007. *Discourse on Method.* **R. Kennington** (trans.) Indianapolis: Focus Publishing. (First published 1637.)

Descartes, R. 1619–/1998. *Regulae ad directionem ingenii / Rules for the Direction of the Natural Intelligence.* **G. Heffernan** (trans.) Amsterdam/Atlanta: Rodopi. (Unfinished work, begun 1619.)

Dreyfus, H. 1992. *What Computers Still Can't Do: A Critique of Artificial Reason.* Cambridge, MA: MIT Press.

Edelman, G. M., G. Tononi. 2000. *A Universe of Consciousness: How Matter Becomes Imagination*. New York: Basic Books.

Eliot, T. S. 1934. *The Rock*. London: Faber & Faber.

Ficocelli, M., J. Terao, G. Nejat. 2015. "Promoting interactions between humans and robots using robotic emotional behavior." *IEEE Transactions on Cybernetics* **46**: 2911–2923.

Frank, M. 1991. *Selbstbewusstsein und Selbsterkenntnis: Essays zur analytischen Philosophie der Subjektivität*. Stuttgart: Reclam.

Freud, S. 1961. "Civilization and its discontents." In J. Strachey (ed.), *Standard Edition of the Works of Sigmund Freud*, Vol. **XXI**. London: Hogarth Press. (First published 1930.) **(pp. 57–146)**.

Fuchs, T. 2019. "The uncanny as atmosphere." In **G. Francesetti, T. Griffero** (eds.) *Psychopathology and Atmospheres: Neither Inside nor Outside*. Cambridge: Cambridge Scholars Publishing (pp. 101–118).

Fuchs, T. 2018. *Ecology of the Brain: The Phenomenology and Biology of the Embodied Mind*. Oxford: Oxford University Press.

Fuchs, T., S. Koch. 2014. "Embodied affectivity: On moving and being moved." In *Frontiers in Psychology* **5**: Article 508.

Galilei, G. 1933. "Il saggiatore." In Antonio Favaro (ed.), *Opere di Galileo Galilei*, Bd. VI. Florenz: G. Barbèra (pp. 204–372).

Gigerenzer, G., P. M. Todd, ABC Research Group. 1999. *Simple Heuristics That Make Us Smart*. New York: Oxford University Press.

Gleick, J. 2011. *The information: A history, a theory, a flood*. New York: Pantheon.

Greenemeier, L. 2010. "Machine self-awareness." *Scientific American* **30**(6): 44–45.

Harari, Y. 2016. *Homo Deus. A Brief History of Tomorrow*. London: Harvill Secker.

Henrich, D. 1970. "Selbstbewusstsein. Kritische Einleitung in eine Theorie." In **R. Bubner** (ed.) *Hermeneutik und Dialektik*. Bd. 1. *Methode und Wissenschaft, Lebenswelt und Geschichte*. Tübingen: Mohr (pp. 257–284).

Hoffmann, E. T. A. 1885. The Sand-Man. J. Y. Bealby (trans.) New York: Charles Scribner's Sons (http://faculty.washington.edu/jdwest/russ430/sandman.pdf).

Hung, L., M. Gregorio, J. Mann, C. Wallsworth, N. Horne, A. Berndt, C. Liu, E. Woldum, A. Au-Yeung, H. Chaudhury. 2019. "Exploring the perceptions of people with dementia about the social robot PARO in a hospital setting." *Dementia* doi: 10.1177/1471301219894141.

Husserl, E. 1991. *On the Phenomenology of the Consciousness of Internal Time*. **John Barnett Brough** (trans.) Dordrecht: Kluwer.

Hustvedt, S. 2016. "The delusions of certainty." In S. Hustvedt: *A Woman Looking at Men Looking at Women: Essays on Art, Sex, and the Mind*. New York: Simon and Schuster (pp. 135–340).

Inkster, B., Sarda, S., Subramanian, V. 2018. "An empathy-driven, conversational Artificial Intelligence agent (Wysa) for digital mental well-being: real-world data evaluation mixed-methods study." *JMIR Mhealth Uhealth* 6(11): e12106.

Janich, P. 2018. *What is Information?* Minnesota: Minnesota University Press.

Kapp, E. 1877. *Grundlinien einer Philosophie der Technik: Zur Entstehungsgeschichte der Cultur aus neuen Gesichtspunkten*. Braunschweig: Westermann.

Jonas, H. 1966. *The Phenomenon of Life: Toward a Philosophical Biology*. New York: Harper & Row.

Kirchner, L., J. Angwin, J. Larson, S. Mattu. 2016. "Machine bias: There's software used across the country to predict future criminals, and it's biased against blacks." *Pro Publica.* https://www.propublica.org/article/machine-bias-risk-assessments-in-criminal-sentencing, last accessed on 01.06.2021.

Klein B., G. Cook. 2012. "Emotional robotics in elder care—a comparison of findings in the UK and Germany." In **S. S. Ge, O. Khatib, J. J. Cabibihan, R. Simmons, M. A. Williams** (eds.) *Social Robotics. ICSR 2012. Lecture Notes in Computer Science.* Berlin, Heidelberg: Springer (pp. 108–117).

Koch, C. 2019. *The Feeling of Life Itself. Why Consciousness Is Widespread but Can't Be Computed.* Cambridge, MA: MIT Press.

Kurzweil, R. 2005. *The Singularity Is Near: When Humans Transcend Biology.* New York: Penguin.

La Mettrie, J. O. de. 1748. *L'Homme Machine.* Leiden: de l'Imp. d'Elie Luzac, fils.

Leibniz, G. W. 1697. "Vorstellung der Binärzahlen, Brief an den Herzog von Braunschweig-Wolfenbüttel Rudolph August, 2. January 1697." *Bibliotheca Augustana* https://www.hs-augsburg.de/~harsch/germanica/Chronologie/17Jh/Leibniz/lei_bina.html, last accessed on 01.06.2021.

Leibniz, G. W. 1890. "Dialogus (August 1677)." In *Philosophische Schriften von Gottfried Wilhelm Leibniz,* Bd. VII. **Hg. von C. I.** (ed.) Gerhardt. Berlin: Weidmannsche Buchhandlung (pp. 190–193).

Leibniz, G. W. 2009. *The Monadology and Other Philosophical Writings.* **R. Latta** (trans.). Ithaca/NY: Cornell University Library. (Monadology first published 1714.) http://home.datacomm.ch/kerguelen/monadology/printable.html.

Manzotti, R., G. Owcarz. 2020. The Ontological Impossibility of Digital Consciousness. *Mind and Matter* 18: 61–72.

Metzinger, T. 1999. *Subjekt und Selbstmodell. Die Perspektivität phänomenalen Bewusstseins vor dem Hintergrund einer naturalistischen Theorie mentaler Repräsentation.* Paderborn: Mentis.

Metzinger, T. 2003. *Being No One: The Self-Model Theory of Subjectivity.* Cambridge/Mass.: MIT Press.

Martín, F., C. Agüero, J. M. Cañas, G. Abella, R. Benítez, S. Rivero, M. Valenti, P Martínez-Martín. 2013. "Robots in therapy for dementia patients." *Journal of Physical Agents* 7: 48–55.

Moor, J. H. 2001. "The status and future of the Turing test." *Minds and Machines* 11(1): 77–93.

Panksepp, J. 1998. *Affective Neuroscience: The Foundations of Human and Animal Emotions.* Oxford, New York: Oxford University Press.

Paul, G. S., E. D. Cox. 1996. *Beyond Humanity: CyberEvolution and Future Minds.* Rockland: Charles River Media.

Pearson, I. 2008. "The future of life. Creating natural, artificial, synthetic and virtual organisms." *European Molecular Biology Organization (EMBO) reports* 9 (Supplement 1): 75–77. doi:10.1038/embor.2008.62

Pinker, S. 1997. *How the Mind Works.* New York: Norton.

Plessner, H. 2019. *Levels of Organic Life and the Human: An Introduction to Philosophical Anthropology.* New York: Fordham University Press. (German original published 1928.)

Salvador, M. J., S. Silver, M. H. Mahoor. 2015. An emotion recognition comparative study of autistic and typically-developing children using the zeno robot. In IEEE (ed.), *International Conference on Robotics and Automation (ICRA)* (pp. 6128–6133). IEEE.

Schummer, J. 2011. *Das Gotteshandwerk. Die künstliche Herstellung von Leben im Labor*. Berlin: Suhrkamp.

Schummers, J., H. Yu, M. Sur. 2008. "Tuned responses of astrocytes and their influence on hemodynamic signals in the visual cortex." *Science* **320** (5883): 1638–1643.

Searle, J. R. 1980. "Minds, brains, and programs." *Behavioral and Brain Sciences* **3**(3): 417–457.

Searle, J. R. 1992. *The Rediscovery of the Mind*. Cambridge, MA: MIT Press.

Searle, J. R. 1998. "How to study consciousness scientifically." *Philosophical Transactions of the Royal Society of London B: Biological Sciences* **353** (1377): 1935–1942.

Shannon, C., W. Weaver. 1964. *The Mathematical Theory of Communication*. Champaign, IL: University of Illinois Press.

Silver, D., J. Schrittwieser, K. Simonyan, I. Antonoglou, A. Huang, A. Guez, T. Hubert, L. Baker, M. Lai, A. Bolton, D. Hassabis. 2017. "Mastering the game of Go without human knowledge." *Nature* **550**(7676): 354–359.

Singer, W. 2009. "Distributed processing and temporal codes in neuronal networks." *Cognitive Neurodynamics* **3**(3): 189–196.

Stoll, J., J. A. Müller, M. Trachsel. 2020. "Ethical issues in online psychotherapy: A narrative review." *Frontiers in Psychiatry* **10**: 993.

Stonier, T. 1999. *Information and the Internal Structure of the Universe*. Berlin, New York: Springer.

Tononi, G., M. Boly, M. Massimini, C. Koch. 2016. "Integrated information theory: From consciousness to its physical substrate." *Nature Reviews Neuroscience* **17**(7): 450–461.

Turkle, S. 2011. *Alone Together: Why We Expect More from Technology and Less from Each Other*. New York: Basic Books.

Turing, A. M. 1950. "Computing machinery and intelligence." *Mind* **59**(October): 433–460.

Varshney, L. R., B. L. Chen, E. Paniagua, D. H. Hall, D. B. Chklovskii. 2011. "Structural properties of the Caenorhabditis elegans neuronal network." *PLoS Computational Biology* **7**(2), e1001066.

Venter, J. C. 2014. *Life at the Speed of Light: From the Double Helix to the Dawn of Digital Life*. London: Penguin.

Weizsäcker, C. F. V. 1974. *Die Einheit der Natur*. München: Deutscher Taschenbuch Verlag.

Wiener, N. 1989. *The Human Use of Human Beings. Cybernetics and Society*. London: Free Association Books. (First published 1950.)

Zahavi, D. 1999. *Self-Awareness and Alterity: A Phenomenological Investigation*. Evanston, IL: Northwestern University Press.

Zolfagharifard, E. 2018. "AI will be 'billions of times' smarter than humans and people must merge with it to survive, claims expert." *Daily Mail Online*, 13 February 2018. https://www.dailymail.co.uk/sciencetech/article-5386255/AI-billions-times-smarter-humans.html, last accessed on 01.06.2021.

Chapter 2

Beyond the Human? A Critique of Transhumanism

It's a burden for us even to be men—men with real, *our own* bodies and blood; we're ashamed of it, we consider it a disgrace, and keep trying to be some unprecedented omni-men. [...] Soon we'll contrive to be born somehow from an idea.

Dostoevsky, Notes from Underground.[1]

Introduction: Between Naturalism and Culturalism

The quotation from Dostoevsky seems prophetic: being an ordinary person made of flesh and blood becomes today more and more a defect. In the face of our machines, we begin to be ashamed of our own imperfection. This seems to presage a fundamental transformation of the previous image of the human, characterized by the following features:

♦ Evolution is understood as a process of progressive differentiation and optimization of life; its outcome, however, is contingent on each point in time. No one intended us to be the way we are. Human nature can no longer be considered as a set constant. It is changeable and available for self-forming.

♦ Humans, in their existing state of development are seen as fundamentally incomplete. The outcome of evolution is only a badly constructed, fallible product, developing blindly.[2] Our perception is prone to all kinds of deceptions and illusions, our thinking is mostly one-sided and distorted by

---

[1] Dostoevsky 1993, 129–30.

[2] For example: "The genetic code also achieves incredible things, but in evolution it was created by trial and error and is therefore poorly structured from an engineering point of view" (Mathwig 2008: 80).

In Defense of the Human Being. Thomas Fuchs, Oxford University Press. © Suhrkamp Verlag 2021. DOI: 10.1093/oso/9780192898197.003.0003

prejudices. Our memories are unreliable, our decisions are highly irrational. Above all, our bodies are fragile, frail, vulnerable, subject to ageing; mortality is the greatest imposition that nature has set upon us. Human nature is therefore not only changeable but *in need* of enhancement—in every respect. We should assume the responsibility for our own further development, rather than—up until now—leave it to blind evolution and chance.

◆ Physical existence is no longer seen primarily as enabling the fulfilment of a life, but increasingly as a restriction of personal freedom. Dependence on bodily preconditions appears to be ever less acceptable; overcoming these becomes the goal of the emancipatory project of modernity. What is propagandized to this end are various forms of body optimization and upgrading, the technological remodeling of human nature, and even the overcoming of death.

Over the last two or three decades, such ideas have become increasingly popular under the heading *transhumanism*, especially in the Anglo-American world. Transhumanists see the opportunity to optimize "inadequate" human nature via bio-, nano-, and computer technologies. Each person should have the right to define and expand his psychic or physical capabilities, his sex, appearance, or intelligence, according to his will (Kurzweil 2005; Bostrom 2009). On another level, transhumanists such as Hans Moravec, Ray Kurzweil, Nick Bostrom, and others predict that we will soon see the fusion of human and machine: cyborgs could form the next stage of evolution and lead us to summits of intelligence and life expectancy unimaginable today. These utopias extend to the fantastic idea of transferring one's own mind to other substrates in the form of pure information ("mind transfer," "mind uploading"). We could then connect our brains to computers, get rid of our aging body of skin and bones completely, and finally attain digital immortality.[3]

Transhumanism thus radicalizes a view of the human body which we have seen is widespread in both life sciences and cultural sciences. It is the conception of the body as an objectifiable vehicle or apparatus that is external to us and is fundamentally subject to our free usage and manipulation. The respective emphases within transhumanism, however, are very different. To put it simply, two positions stand opposed to one another:

a) The *naturalistic position* assumes a biological determinacy of the human being: genes, hormones and neurons control the development of our personality, our moods, our social behavior—even moral attitudes such as altruism

---

[3] "If humans can merge their minds with computers, why would they not discard the human form and become an immortal being?" (Paul & Cox 1996: 21).

can be traced back to what is advantageous in terms of evolutionary survival. Attachment, love, or trust are only epiphenomena of biochemical processes or organic algorithms. The biosciences clarify the mechanisms of these determinations with the aim of taking their control into our own hands. Ritalin, oxytocin, mood enhancers, stimulants, or neuro-enhancers are the means available today to put us into desired states or moods. Oxytocin as a prosocial hormone is currently a central object of research into the treatment of empathy deficits or even relationship conflicts (Ditzen et al. 2009; Hurlemann et al. 2010). In psychiatry, "deep brain stimulation" methods are also playing an increasingly important role, for example in treatment of severe depression or obsessive-compulsive disorders.

b) By contrast, the *culturalist-voluntarist position* assumes that there is or should be no biological determination of the individual. Intelligence, personality, gender, and other characteristics of the physical constitution should ultimately only be based on cultural socialization and social constructions. A predetermined nature of the body is either disputed, or at least seen as an undesirable limitation of the individual's freedom to redesign themself. As a man or woman, one is not born but made, and this would also give the freedom to determine one's own gender. The consequences range all the way to utopian-transhumanist positions that praise the overcoming of our physical nature as the completion of the emancipatory project of modernity.

Both positions, as different as they are, are ultimately based on the same premise, namely a dualistic opposition of body and mind. This dualism is interpreted in the one case as the complete determination of the mind *by the body*, while in the other case it serves as the starting point for a radical voluntarism of the *mind* in relation to the body.[4] Paradoxically, both positions lead to similar consequences, namely the demand for ever more extensive manipulations of one's own physical nature. A paradigmatic reference can be made to Donna Haraway's "Cyborg Manifesto" (1985/1995): for her, the metaphor of the cyborg stands for a radical feminist overthrow of traditional gender identities and the concept of human nature:

> By the late twentieth century [...] we are all chimeras, theorized and fabricated hybrids of machine and organism; in short, we are cyborgs. The cyborg is our ontology. (Haraway 1991: 1)

....

[4] It is worth noting that both radical biologism and radical voluntarism were already realized in the totalitarian systems of the twentieth century: in National Socialism under the slogan of a "struggle for existence" and at least hinted at in Nietzsche's "blond beast" (1988: 275), in the *Manifesto of the Communist Party* in the demand for a "new socialist man" who frees himself from all natural conditions and limitations.

We currently find the same idea in functionalist theories, according to which the human mind has not only the brain as its substrate, but also external prostheses, memory stores, and data systems—we are, in the words of philosopher Andy Clark, already *Natural-Born Cyborgs* (2003). There is nothing to prevent the mixing of technology and body, since our physical nature itself is already conceived by analogy with a technical system.[5]

Neither position, however, in their dualistic one-sidedness, do justice to the anthropological basic structure, namely our *embodiment*. Humans, so I will argue in the following, are neither biological machines nor pure minds, they are first and foremost living, bodily beings. Being bodily is not something external to us, it is rather the foundation of our existence, precisely because all feeling, perception, thought, and action is a form of our embodied enactment of life. At the same time, of course, humans are beings with the ability to take stances towards their corporeality, that is, to form an instrumental relationship with their body. But they can thereby neither ignore their corporeality nor annul it. Rather, they must form, cultivate, and integrate it into their ideas of a good life. Humans are therefore at once biological and cultural beings: the cultural shaping of their own bodily nature is part of their anthropological structure.[6]

---

[5] This corresponds to an increasingly widespread culture of technical self-monitoring, also known as "quantified self": It involves digital self-tracking through pulse monitors, pedometers, fitness and sleep trackers, calorie apps and other means that incorporate data acquisition into daily life, often with the goal of improving physical and mental performance (see Lupton 2016). The self-reification is obvious: Not your own body perception, but the apparatus now tells you how you feel.

[6] At this point, a comment is needed on the traditionally problematic relationship between "nature" and "culture." The fact that, already in prehistoric times, the cultural development of the human being had a retroactive effect on its natural evolution may be considered as certain. For example, the lowering of the human larynx in comparison with that of other primates can be explained primarily by the fact that it allows the formation of more differentiated linguistic sounds (see Lieberman 2006: 246 ff., Lieberman et al. 2007). Since in other respects lowering the larynx has certain *disadvantages* (namely the incomplete separation of air and food ways, with the danger of asphyxiation), the development of linguistic communication and the corresponding genetic evolution of our speech tools must have favored each other. The evolution of nature and culture in humans can therefore not be separated from each other.

This insight dynamizes the traditional opposition between "nature" and "culture" but does not completely eliminate the concept of nature. This is because the ontogenetic cultivation of human embodiment, which through habitualization turns into our "second nature," takes place on quite different time scales than the phylogenetic changes in human genetics. In this respect, despite the entanglement of cultural and natural evolution and despite the interaction of cultural history and second nature, we are justified in speaking of a biological or "*first*" nature of *Homo sapiens sapiens*, which has remained largely constant

However, this relationship to one's own corporeality also opens up the possibility of its radical, i.e., organic change. And the fact that the course of evolution has produced the human organism *in this precise form* is of course not enough to justify it. Such an attempt would be subject to the well-known "naturalistic fallacy," i.e., to infer from *being* like this that it *should* be like this. Who would deny us the path of transhuman progress that would make today's humans—seen from the future perfect of the "new man"—appear as mere distant ancestors, not unlike our rather amused look back on *Homo erectus* or *Australopithecus*?

As soon as the idea of a divine order of creation has lost its general validity, the constancy and binding character of human nature is called into question. The question must be answered in a different way. The defense of human nature that I will undertake in the following—nature understood as the biological constitution that currently characterizes *Homo sapiens*—rests essentially on three arguments:

1) Can human nature be improved at all? This question may seem surprising, however imperfect and deficient in physical, cognitive, emotional, or moral features the constitution of *Homo sapiens* may appear. On closer inspection, however, it will become clear that it is not so simple, because every supposed improvement disturbs the proportions of human assets. In other words: improvements would have their price, a price greater than first appears—and one would have to be prepared to pay it.

2) In its revolutionary variant, i.e., the fundamental genetic or technological transformation of the body, transhumanism becomes *posthumanism*, and thus self-contradictory: because it abolishes the basis from which this self-transformation could appear meaningful in the first place. Because notions of the good, which every enhancement or reengineering of human nature are ultimately intended to serve, are themselves still tied to the natural basis of *Homo sapiens*. "Beyond the human" cannot be a meaningful goal of our striving—unless the goal is merely to abolish the present human being.

3) Finally, in its radical-dualist variant—mind transfer or mind uploading—transhumanism rests on a false concept of consciousness. The human mind is not an ensemble of digitizable algorithms and information but constitutively alive and embodied. Selfhood or personal identity cannot therefore

---

over the last 100,000 years. In the following, this concept of nature is also meant when discussing possible "improvements" of human nature—whatever such improvements might be. The fact that transhumanists often do not differentiate clearly enough here and already count individual enhancements (e.g., the use of psychostimulants, mood enhancers etc.) as "improvement of the human being" does not change the fact that these are two categorically different forms of optimization.

be represented as data sets. Even if this variant of transhumanism seems particularly abstruse, it is worth refuting it, not least in view of the difference between human and artificial intelligence.

But before I elaborate on these arguments, I would like to take a look at the history of ideas of the perfection or transgression of the human being, against the background of which current transhumanism is to be seen. Granted, if one places it in this tradition, one does it too much honor, because in Thomas Aquinas, Rousseau, or Nietzsche, for example, this tradition achieved a depth of insight that is in no way matched by the shallow utopias of a biological optimization of man. Nevertheless, it is at least worth taking a look at this tradition, since it is only in such contrasts that it becomes clear how far the great idea of human perfection has fallen today.

The Idea of Perfectibility

The concept of the cultural, intellectual, and moral *perfectibility* of man, first formulated around the middle of the eighteenth century by Rousseau, has a long history. Christianity already knew the ideal of perfection in the imitation of God: "Be perfect, as the Father in heaven is perfect" (Matthew 5:48). Paul calls on the Ephesians to cast off the "old man" and to put on the "new man," created in the image of God (Eph 4:24). In Augustine, and later in Thomas Aquinas, the idea that man is the being in which nature transcends itself towards the divine is found only in anticipation of eternal life.[7] On the other hand there is the doctrine of original sin as the inherent infirmity of human nature, which can only be completely overcome eschatologically.

In Dante's *Paradise* (2007) the poet describes the transformation and purification he experiences in his ascent with Beatrice through the spheres by means of a neologism *"trasumanar"*—from *trans* and *humanus*, i.e., "going beyond the human" (Canto I: 70). "Man infinitely transcends man," Pascal later writes in his *Pensées* (Pascal 1995: 35): human nature in its fundamental brokenness will not be the final word in the history of salvation. Instead, the demand to already imitate on earth Christ as the model of highest human perfection (*"ecce homo"*) is constitutive of the Christian idea of salvation.

---

[7] Thomas is concerned here with perfect bliss *(beatitudo)* as the highest goal laid out in human nature. Nevertheless, humans cannot reach that goal by their natural gifts alone, not even by reason, but only in the *"beatitudo supernaturalis,"* which the vision of God grants us (STh I-II: q 5, a 5, co; Thomas Aquinas 2008). One could also say: by means of God's grace, humans, transcending their nature, first bring this nature to itself.

With the Renaissance, the idea of humans' freedom to shape their own lives in this world came into view for the first time, even if this freedom is still given to him by God himself. In Pico della Mirandola's treatise *De hominis dignitate* (1486) God speaks to man:

> The nature of all other things is limited and constrained within the bounds of laws prescribed by me: thou, coerced by no necessity, shalt ordain for thyself the limits of thy nature in accordance with thine own free will, in whose hand I have placed thee. [...] I have made thee neither of heaven nor of earth, neither mortal nor immortal, so that thou mayest with greater freedom of choice and with more honor, as though the maker and molder of thyself, fashion thyself in whatever shape thou shalt prefer. (Pico della Mirandola 1486/1942: 348)

Here, the idea of a self-transgression of humanity is set forth which no longer follows a plan of salvation but is subject to his own freedom and creative potency. In a world determined by nature, it is given to humans alone to shape and change themselves according to their own will. "Man is the first liberated being of creation," Herder will later say (1784–1785/1967: 146). *Bildung* (education, self-formation) takes the place of mere likeness to God. The *humanum* becomes self-determination, but thus also a problem—an experiment of history that can succeed or fail. "If man was created for freedom and has no law on earth other than the one he lays down for himself, he must become the most savage creature if he does not soon recognize the law of God in nature," warns Herder (Herder 1967: 16).

This ambivalence of our human freedom to form ourselves is also inherent in Rousseau's concept of "*perfectibilité*," by which he defines the essential difference between man and animal (Rousseau 1755/2011): the human is a phylogenetically and ontogenetically open, malleable and in principle infinitely perfectible being. Only culture and education let humans come to themselves; all our achievements are derived from this. But it is also the same development that moves us further and further away from nature; it is the source of inequality and thus of the misfortune that civilization produces. Perfectibility, therefore, contains the possibility of emancipation as well as alienation, and it remains to be seen which of the two will eventually prevail.

In the further course of the Enlightenment, however, perfectibility was understood in a much more optimistic way. In his *Esquisse d'un tableau historique des progrès de l'esprit Humain* (1794), Condorcet expressed his conviction

> that there has been set no limit to the perfection of human abilities; that the perfectibility of man is really indefinite; that the progress of this perfectibility [...] has its limit only in the duration of the planet onto which nature has thrown us. (Condorcet 1794/ 1822, 3–4; my trans.)

The history of salvation has unmistakably transformed itself into an inner-worldly history of progress. Here the possibility of *biological* perfectibility appears for the first time:

> [...] and yet so far we have only assumed the same natural abilities, the same organization, which man already has. How great would be [...] the extent of his hopes, if one could believe that these natural abilities themselves, this organization, are also susceptible to improvement [...] (Condorcet 1794: 303–4)

Condorcet's vision would take on more concrete form with Darwin's theory of inheritance and evolution. Perfectibility first became a common historical-philosophical concept in the nineteenth century, seeming to be sufficiently justified by the progress of science and technology, the abolition of slavery and the general humanization of living conditions. The actual self-transgression of humanity to a new, future being is found for the first time again with Karl Marx, namely, as Karl Löwith notes, with unmistakable borrowings from Christian eschatology and apocalypticism: the messianic, redemptive function of the proletariat as "chosen people" and germ cell of the new man is just as much a part of his theory as the antagonism of bourgeoisie and proletariat, in analogy to the final struggle between Christ and the Antichrist (Löwith 1953: 48).

With the Russian Revolution this leads to the utopia of the socialist "New Man," in its boldest form proposed by Leon Trotsky:

> Man will make it his purpose to master his own feelings, to raise his instincts to the heights of consciousness, to make them transparent, [...] and thereby to raise himself to a new plane, to create a higher social biologic type, or, if you please, a superman. [...] The average human type will rise to the heights of an Aristotle, a Goethe, or a Marx. And above this ridge new peaks will rise. (Trotsky 1924/2005: 264)

In contrast to this, Nietzsche's idea of the superman, as is well known, has a completely different character—not the collective realization of the human species-essence but the aristocratic growth of the "will to power" (Nietzsche 1980a: 146f.), the elevation of the supreme individual above the herd man. "*I teach you the superman.* Man is something that is to be overcome"—thus begins Nietzsche's *Zarathustra* (Nietzsche 1980a: 14). Man's self-transgression is at the same time the answer to the loss of transcendence, the death of God. Now that the world no longer strives for a divine final purpose, the superman becomes the bearer of the revaluation of all values (29–31), the object of his own creative self-perfection, which lets him also accept the "eternal return of the same" as redeeming insight (271–277). This transformation can take place as self-cultivation, but also—this is where the new theory of evolution comes into play—as breeding, as Nietzsche indicates in the following passage:

> One question keeps coming back to me, a tempting and terrible question perhaps: […] Would it not be time, the more the type "herd animal" is now being developed in Europe, to make an attempt with a fundamental, artificial and conscious *breeding* of the opposite type and its virtues? (Nietzsche 1980b: 73)

In any case, the superman can create himself—be it through self-education, self-improvement, or even through biological mutation.

Both Marx and Nietzsche thus reinterpreted the Christian-eschatological self-transcendence of man, albeit in very different ways. What they have in common is the transformation of the history of salvation into a radical inner-worldly utopia. The twentieth century has, of course, brought to light the potentially totalitarian core of the idea of the "new man"—even if the connecting lines to the utopias of the nineteenth century cannot be drawn too directly.[8]

If this idea is resurrected in the crude materialism and naive technical optimism of transhumanists, one might be reminded of Marx's statement that all historical events occur twice, first as tragedy, then as farce (Marx 1852/1960: 115). But we do not yet know what the real consequences of the present utopias of human betterment will be. At the very least, they are renewed evidence that a striving for self-transgression seems to be inherent in man—so that with the loss of eschatological transcendence, even a trans- or posthuman self-abolition of the species may gain attraction. Humans do not seem to be able to live well with themselves.

The transhumanism to which I am returning has its origins in the more radical posthumanism of the 1980s.[9] It begins with a futuristic glorification of technology and the vision of a posthuman machine age, as in Hans Moravec's *Mind Children: The Future of Robot and Human Intelligence* (1988):

---

[8] The religious roots of the totalitarian ideologies of the 20th century have been examined above all by Eric Voegelin (1939; 1968). In his view, they represent secularized late forms of the basic patterns of religious stories of decay and redemption, whose messianic as well as apocalyptic motifs are now projected into history.

[9] In general, transhumanism seeks only to improve the present human being, while posthumanism criticizes anthropocentrism more fundamentally and even envisages our replacement by a new species. However, the two tendencies cannot be strictly separated. Sorgner (2010) mentions as a possible criterion for a posthuman being the loss of the ability to mate with humans, comparable to the incompatibility between humans and chimpanzees; it would therefore amount to a new biological (or biotechnological) species. Bostrom, on the other hand, defines post-humanity quite arbitrarily in that at least one of the following characteristics must be present: (a) life expectancy of more than 500 years, (b) cognitive abilities that are more than two standard deviations above the current human maximum, (c) extensive control over one's own sensory perceptions, (d) extensive disappearance of mental suffering (Bostrom 2009: 204).

> What awaits us is […] a future, which, from our present vantage point, is best de-
> scribed by the words "postbiological" or even "supernatural". It is a world in which the
> human race has been swept away by the tide of cultural change, usurped by its own
> artificial progeny. […] within the next century, they [the machines] will mature into
> entities as complex as ourselves, and eventually into something transcending every-
> thing we know – in whom we can take pride when they refer to themselves as our des-
> cendants. (Moravec 1988: 1)

Moravec also already formulated the idea of digital immortality through "trans-
migration" of the spirit, which according to his estimate should technically be
possible as early as 2018 (Moravec 1988: 108). While biological humanity is
slowly dying out, humans will ensure the continued existence of their minds
through computer simulation. Moravec's successor Ray Kurzweil has mean-
while corrected the prognosis: he doesn't expect the singularity, the fusion of
human and computer into a cyborg and thus digital immortality, before 2045
(Kurzweil 2005). Yet the idea of mind uploading remains the same:

> Up until now, our mortality was tied to the longevity of our hardware. When the hard-
> ware crashed, that was it […] As we cross the divide to instantiate ourselves into our
> computational technology, our identity will be based on our evolving mind file. We will
> be software, not hardware. (Kurzweil 1999: 128f.)

However, the more moderate transhumanist movement is no longer focused
only on a post-human age but is dedicated to all variants of optimizing human
nature that could be achieved with biotechnological means in the near future.
This, too, could gradually lead to a "Homo optimus" as praised by the Oxford
futurologist Ian Pearson:

> With optimized genomes and bodies enhanced by links to external technology, people
> could be more beautiful … more intelligent, more emotionally sophisticated, more
> physically able, more socially connected, generally healthier and happier all round.
> (Pearson, quoted in Griffiths 2016)[10]

One may consider these and similar promises to be too superficial and foolish
to take seriously. But the transhumanist utopias are now too widespread to be
simply ignored. And thought experiments on the transformation of human

---

[10] Let us quote another description of future transhumanistic pleasures: "You have just cele-
brated your 170th birthday and you feel stronger than ever. Each day is a joy. You have
invented entirely new art forms, which exploit the new kinds of cognitive capacities
and sensibilities you have developed. You still listen to music – music that is to Mozart
what Mozart is to bad Muzak. You are communicating with your contemporaries using
a language that has grown out of English over the past century and that has a vocabulary and expressive power that enables you to share and discuss thoughts and feelings that
unaugmented humans could not even think or experience […] Things are getting better,
but already each day is fantastic" (Bostrom 2008: 112).

nature may have a virtue: by pointing out the contradictions and aporias into which such ideas lead, they may ultimately contribute to reconciling us with the imperfections of human existence. For this reason, I now turn to the arguments mentioned at the beginning.[11]

Can Human Nature be Improved?

Let us begin with the question of whether human nature could be fundamentally improved by genetic, neuro-technical, or other interventions. This does not refer to technical means to *restore or substitute* bodily functions, such as all forms of prostheses, implants or brain-computer connections, for example in the case of paralysis. Likewise, I will leave aside here all *temporary increases* in bodily functions by pharmacological or technical means (mood elevators, cognitive enhancers, stimulants, or neuromodulation). Although they too must be subjected to an ethical evaluation, this is not of a fundamental, i.e., anthropological nature, but will have to be based primarily on individual side effects or social consequences (for example, the unequal distribution of the necessary resources, a possible "race to the top," etc.). Here, I only consider conceivable permanent interventions in *human nature*. Would there at least be the possibility of a better version of *Homo sapiens*—a biotechnologically revolutionized "*Homo optimus*"?

Cognitive Skills

Let us start with cognitive enhancement, i.e., the increase in vigilance, attention, learning, and memory performance, as is already possible with psychostimulants such as methylphenidate, modafinil or amphetamines. Transcranial neurostimulation is also increasingly used to promote learning performance (Kuo & Nitsche 2012; Krause & Kadosh 2013). However, only a *universal* increase in human cognitive performance among the entire population would avoid the problem of injustice which would immediately arise with *individual* enhancement (many apparent advantages of neuro-enhancement would, of course, quickly lapse if everyone were to benefit from it). So, let us ask ourselves: would the universal (i.e., not only situative and selective) enhancement of the previously mentioned abilities really be desirable?

At first glance, an *increase in attention span* seems to be an undeniable advantage, if we are dealing with speed of learning or professional efficiency. But attention is a scarce resource, and many stimuli and possible objects compete

---

[11] See also the contributions of Hauskeller (2011, 2014), one of the most important critics of transhumanism, arguing in a similar direction.

for it. An excessive focusing of attention can lead to the exclusion of other objects which are possibly also useful. Patients taking Ritalin, a psychostimulant used to treat attention deficit disorder, report that the increased fixation on the respective task renders everything else secondary. Cognitive focusing increases but the patient's need for interpersonal relationships reduces, along with interest in new experiences, spontaneity and creativity.[12] An increased ability to focus may undoubtedly be an advantage in certain situations; however, a general enhancement of human attention capacity would come at the price of a loss of openness, flexibility, and susceptibility for novelty. Instead, the already existing spiral of increased performance, acceleration, and competition would be intensified. So, do we want to function better and better—or remain flexible, open, and creative? With this enhancement we are faced with a typical conflict of optimization—one which characterizes all other purported enhancements.

The same is true, for example, for the increase in memory performance. The ability to remember much or everything seems self-evidently to be desirable, and in many cases, it is. But whoever memorizes everything can no longer *forget* anything. The vital balance between remembering and forgetting is easily lost from view. Forgetting relieves the memory of an overabundance of details, so that the really meaningful memories can come to the fore in the first place. William James already pointed this out:

> Selection is the very keel on which our mental ship is built. And in this case of memory its utility is obvious. If we remembered everything, we should on most occasions be as ill off as if we remembered nothing. (James 1890/1950: 680)

Forgetting also allows us to process and discard what we have experienced, thus neutralizing the potentially paralyzing effect of the past, which would otherwise continue to grow in life. Only in this way does the mind receive the possibility for renewal, the ability to see the world again and again with new eyes.

The importance of this balance can be seen in a rare anomaly, namely *hyperthymesia*. Although people with this syndrome can use their overdeveloped memory to trace every day of their lives in minute detail, they are also exposed to a constant crossfire of mostly trivial memories that they cannot suppress.[13] In addition, the over-specific memory makes it difficult to think in terms of concepts. As Lurija (2000) describes it, for those affected there is no

---

[12] On this topic see Swartwood et al. (2003), Mohamed (2014); Fallon et al. (2017);, and Gvirts et al. (2017).

[13] As hyperthymesiac Jill Price writes in her autobiography: "As I grew up and more and more memories were stored in my brain, more and more of them flashed through my mind in this endless barrage, and I became a prisoner to my memory" (Price 2008: 3). Another description is given by a patient of Lurija: "Memories are popping into my head randomly all

"tree" per se, just as there is no general "oak" or "beech," but always only this singular, very specific beech behind the house, while the beech in the forest appears to them as a completely different tree, incomparable to the first one. So, if you can't forget a single detail, you can't abstract either and literally can't see the wood for the trees.[14]

Forgetting thus has a liberating effect in many ways; indeed, in the end, remembering and forgetting *make each other possible*, just like foreground and background. Therefore, if the mere maximization of memory is not a real advantage but a danger, any meaningful enhancement should allow one to select memories according to whether one wants to keep or forget them. But, even if such a selection were technically possible at all, the question would still remain as to what it should depend on—the relevance of memories is constantly changing, and it may well be that we would like to reverse the choice at a later point in time. It is precisely the characteristic of our memory that it creates a lively balance between remembering and forgetting, which is constantly reconfigured according to current requirements—the seemingly forgotten can unexpectedly reappear in suitable situations. In contrast, a targeted deletion or, conversely, the generation of memories through brain stimulation would put an artificial identity in the place of one's own life story. Such a memory design may be attractive to transhumanists, but most people will shy away from such a possibility. Authenticity is still an important value for us.

Happiness and Morality

Let us move on to improving *mood*. Who could blame people for wanting to give pharmacological or technological support to their experience of happiness in the face of the hardships and manifold frustrations of life? But well-being, contentment, and happiness are in a sense the rewards that nature has provided for us, the return on labor and effort, and they are usually in proportion to the effort invested. Mountain hikers know the difference in the experience of happiness when they have climbed a peak themselves or when they have taken the

---

the time, as though there is a screen in my head playing scenes from movies of years of my life that have been spliced into one another, hopping around from day to day, year to year, the good, the bad, the joyful, and the devastating, without my conscious control" (Lurija 2000: 33; my trans.).

[14] Similarly, in his story "Funes el Memorioso" ("Funes the Memorious"), Jorge Louis Borges depicts a hyperthymesiac who had learned English, French, Portuguese, and Latin without effort, but who "was not very capable of thought. To think is to forget differences, generalize, make abstractions. In the teeming world of Funes, there were only details, almost immediate in their presence" (Borges 1962a: 115).

cable car to the top. Any intense *joie de vivre* is the fruit of reaching real goals, and it is usually proportional to the resistance on the way there.[15]

If well-being and happiness were to be kept at a permanently high level, so to speak free of charge, not only would the human striving for self-development and self-transgression slacken, the experience of happiness would also flatten, since it would come about "undeservedly" and not as a satisfying result of one's own efforts. At the same time, tolerance of frustration would diminish, as we would lose practice in overcoming obstacles and setbacks. On the other hand, were well-being to be gradually increased, actual individual and social griev-ances could go unperceived or be accepted indifferently, instead of our fighting against them. All this resembles the changes which may be observed in long-term drug addicts. Let us finally think of Huxley's *Brave New World* (1932), where the consumption of the mood-lifting drug "soma" provides the popula-tion with a sedative, flat pleasure: such an enhancement seems hardly desirable, even if it were a voluntary measure and not decreed by the state.[16]

A completely different variant of proposals aims at improving the *sociality and morality* of the human being. Persson and Savulescu (2012), for example, argue that the very prospect of cognitive enhancement would be potentially dangerous if it were not accompanied by an increase in the willingness to feel altruistic and to act pro-socially. This is because the evolutionary endowment of the human being, they argue, is only oriented towards relationships in small groups and towards the immediate future but is psychologically and morally insufficient for coping with global tasks and handling dangerous technologies. Since characteristics such as altruism or a sense of justice have a biological

---

[15] It is no coincidence that the centers in the brain relevant to the experience of satisfac-tion and happiness (limbic system, *nucleus accumbens*) are called "reward systems." From a neurobiological point of view, the desire and the prospect of reward are of central import-ance for the motivation to act, for curiosity, and the striving for success. Of course, this does not sufficiently explain human striving; it would be grotesque to assume that Beethoven, van Gogh, or Kafka were primarily concerned with creating well-being or pleasure through their work. However, since the messenger substances of the reward system (dopamine, endorphins) are also released when a person consumes drugs, for example, or indulges in gambling, an addiction can develop instead of a healthy motivation to act. The feeling of pleasure is then sought directly, no longer on the path to overcoming real resistance.

[16] Of course, in the course of a universal enhancement, it could happen that more and more people prefer the pharmacologically or technologically generated pleasure to the satisfac-tion that follows effort. Even now, many people prefer to use the lift to reach a summit, and certainly that is their right. Nevertheless, a general tendency towards effortless enjoyment would most probably lead to all the concomitant symptoms of addiction. This is when the question of the image of man that underlies such optimization efforts becomes a polit-ical one.

basis, it is ethically indispensable to optimize such moral dispositions pharmacologically or genetically (see also Lavazza & Reichlin 2019 for an overview).

For example, the hormone oxytocin can increase people's confidence, empathy, and bonding tendency. Couldn't this be used to make it easier for people who are unwilling to bond to form relationships, or indeed could it make it easier for the whole of humanity to do so? The neurotransmitter serotonin also promotes pro-social behavior and increases aversion to inflicting violence on others. This was investigated in a study on the well-known "trolley dilemma": a tram threatens to roll over five people on a track; is it possible to save these five people by diverting the tram to another track where it would only kill one person? A pharmacological increase in serotonin levels in test subjects lead them to develop an increased emotional resistance to induced killing (i.e., diverting the tram) and to engaging in rational-utilitarian calculations (Crocket et al. 2010). Would serotonin therefore be a suitable moral enhancer?

The last example in particular shows that there is no general consensus on moral dilemmas—utilitarians would indignantly reject the increase in serotonin as a promotion of "irrational" moral perceptions. Moreover, here too, a one-sided promotion of moral dispositions is always accompanied by adverse consequences elsewhere. If oxytocin makes people more relationship-oriented, they are also more willing to accept disadvantages in the relationship, even to let themselves be dominated by others, to their detriment. It has been shown that exposure to oxytocin also tends to favor members of one's own group over strangers; it even promotes prejudice and xenophobia (De Dreu et al. 2010, 2011). The neurochemically increased sense of attachment thus remains focused on the core group, quite contrary to the universalistic morality hoped for by Persson and Savulescu. And when people become more aggression-inhibited by serotonin or other means, this may at first sight favor a more peaceful world, but it may also give free rein to criminals or psychopaths who are only out to manipulate others. Already, in the "ultimatum game," another test procedure to determine the mutual fairness of the participants, serotonin increases individuals' willingness to accept unfair offers from the other side (Crocket et al. 2010). An increased inhibition of aggression would thus be a double-edged sword, and it could turn out that a world optimized with serotonin would by no means look more peaceful but in fact more authoritarian and violent than one had imagined.

Thus, the aporia of a moral improvement of the human being becomes clear: there are no moral dispositions that can be affirmed without reservation, since here the good or the appropriate for the human being consists essentially in a balance of contradictory requirements, i.e., in a *proportionality* that at least attempts to reconcile the unavoidable contradictions of the *conditio humana*.

Aging and Death

A final issue on which the prevailing biotechnological utopias set their sights is ageing and death. Progress in bio-gerontology, in particular the discovery of genes that control the ageing process, has given impetus to visions of halting the ageing of the body and extending life ever further, possibly even achieving immortality. "To abolish the greatest evil: death," demands Max More (1990: 10), one of the founders of the transhumanist movement, and if guaranteed immortality is not quite the goal, then at least a life span no longer limited by aging.[17] Against the objection that we might get bored in the face of eternity, transhumanists Nick Bostrom and Rebecca Roache list a number of attractive projects that could then be realized, such as learning to play all the instruments in an orchestra, writing a book in a major language, or traveling to Alpha Centauri: "if we could reasonably expect from an early age to live indefinitely, we could embark on projects designed to keep us occupied for hundreds or thousands of years" (Bostrom & Roache 2007: 126).

But immortality is a contradictory concept, because examined more closely, death is as much a part of life as night is of day. Let us first consider the basic conditions of life: organisms maintain themselves and their internal order in the face of entropy, the disordered processes of the physical environment. This "improbable" order (negative entropy) is, however, dependent in principle on the exchange of matter and energy with the environment and thus always remains precarious: living beings are needy and therefore mortal. The loss of inner homeostasis means their downfall. Life must therefore constantly be wrested from the threat of decay, as it were; it is in principle exposed to the possibility of death. All living beings can die, and from the stage of multicellular organisms onwards death is their certain fate.

But this confrontation with possible not-being also means, as Hans Jonas (1992) emphasized, the *self-affirmation* of the living being. And this is simultaneously the basis for everything that represents a value or good in the world. Because it is the significance for one's own continued existence that makes things and conditions attractive, desirable or else painful and threatening. Desire and pain, need and satisfaction have their meaning, their reason, in the

---

[17] "If immortality should not be a goal, indefinitely long lifespan can be" (More 2009). What is meant is this: although death would no longer inevitably occur due to aging and disintegration of the organism, it would still be a contingent possibility, namely due to external causes such as accidents, homicide, or suicide. Therefore, despite a lifespan that is unlimited in principle, at some point death would in all probability occur. A *necessary* immortality (i.e., the de facto complete invulnerability) is certainly beyond what is conceivable for living beings.

fact that life must assert itself against possible death. The threat of not being, the sting of death, is what elicits the affirmation of life and its value. The lust for life therefore has the fear of death as its necessary complement.

This applies first to the basic conditions of life; but it also corresponds to our existential experience. Only with the consciousness of death does the appreciation of life grow; only "being towards death" (Heidegger) gives life its actual seriousness. "Teach us to count our days so that we may gain a wise heart," say the Psalms (90:12). "Anyone who taught men to die would teach them how to live," writes Montaigne in the same spirit in his *Essais* (I, 20; 1993: 28). People who have been close to death or suffer from a terminal illness find the time remaining all the more precious, and their experience of the present becomes more intense. What then would it mean if a lifetime were no longer limited? The experiences of happiness, intensity, and presence would surely be flattened out, since the colors of life shine only against the dark background of death. Certainly, desire would still stand out from pain, joy, from suffering. But all pleasures would be repeatable as often as desired and would be already devalued by this.

In another of Jorge Louis Borges' tales, "The Immortal," the journey to the immortal troglodytes leads the narrator to the realization that endless life means paralysis in the eternal return of the same—it amounts to extreme boredom (Borges 1981a). After having drunk the water of eternal life, the narrator becomes more and more apathetic, losing all interest in himself and the world, because nothing is of any importance anymore.

> Everything among the mortals has the value of the irretrievable and the perilous. Among the immortals, on the other hand, every act (and every thought) is the echo of others that preceded it in the past, with no visible beginning […] There is nothing that is not as if lost in a maze of indefatigable mirrors. Nothing can happen only once, nothing is preciously precarious. (Borges 1962b: 146)

With an infinite lifetime, everything remains possible and everything reversible. So, there is no *decision* in the existential sense any more. Today I can do A instead of B, but it remains without seriousness and urgency, because next time I could choose the alternative. Nothing would impel us any more to use our time wisely, to realize plans, even to find ourselves. Life would ripple away, ever further, without end, but also without goal.[18]

One might object that it would be sufficient to at least increase the life span to two or three hundred years. How many more life possibilities could be realized

---

[18] From the perspective of identity theory, Bernard Williams (2010) in particular has argued that immortal life would inevitably lead to monotony and eternal boredom.

then, what skills could still be learned, talents be used, projects be realized? But one forgets that such an extension may seem welcome only from the perspective of our current life expectancy. Once human life expectancy has averaged 300 years, the individuals' view of their achievements and their goals will surely adapt to the new lifespan and they will feel it to be as limited as our current 80 or 90 years. And is it really true that the value of experience and the realization of projects lies in their mere addition? Does the success of human life consist in the quantity of happiness achieved? Doesn't the effort to maximize the return on one's life, in the manner of *homo economicus*, seem rather detrimental to a fulfilled life?

But there is something else: any prolongation of life, and even more so immortality, would upset the balance between the generations to the detriment of our descendants. From a biological point of view, the death of individuals is already the prerequisite for creating space for new life and thus, in the course of evolution, for new variants of life. With their reproduction, living beings have realized this principle. Their continued survival would only lead to overpopulation and would rapidly consume the ecological resources of their offspring. The overpopulation of the earth by humans is already obvious—just imagine the exploitation of resources by immortal or nearly immortal humans; what wars for land and resources we would have to expect!

A similar problem concerns intergenerational relations. Ultimately, mortality is the precondition of the "natality" of the human being, whose fundamental significance Hannah Arendt (1951/1976) already demonstrated. For her, natality is the source of the new, the promise and the future; it means being able to see the world again and again with new eyes and to decide freely, without being determined by a fateful past. But this new beginning, which every child's coming into the world signifies, is in an emphatic sense only possible when his or her elders depart the world. Otherwise, the younger generations would never have room for their own heyday; they would never be freed from the gerontocracy of their ancestors. The existing problems of the aging of Western societies would multiply.

Death is still the most effective limitation of our tendency to egocentricity and narcissism. We pass life on to others and care for their future, not just our own. If our striving is not driven by the will to leave a better world for our children and grandchildren, it revolves around itself and becomes directionless. If human beings were immortal, their willingness to produce offspring and promote their future would also quickly diminish. Mankind would continue to age, would freeze in its well-established forms of life, and finally, in the repetition of the ever same, would succumb to an all-overshadowing exhaustion.

Lastly, the dissolution of the lifespan would also have serious consequences for the natality and spontaneity of the individual. The weight of the past, of what has already been lived and known, of acquired attitudes and habits would continue to increase. Unlike physical ageing, mental ageing could not be stopped, namely the loss of the malleability of the personality, openness to new things, flexibility, and creativity, which are usually a privilege of youth. At the same time, the longer one lives in the ever-present world, the more one becomes a stranger—as old people are already experiencing today in an ever more rapidly changing society. Of course, one could imagine, as Jonas (1992) writes, that future bioengineers would not only free life from the burdensome side-effects of aging, but would also ensure that old memories were regularly erased. This would have the consequence, however, that the continuity of personal identity would be fragmented or completely interrupted. We would thus have the choice of either living more and more in our own past, or of living in an ever-new present without personal continuity.

If we keep all this realistically in mind, the utopia of immortality begins to become less attractive after all. There is no doubt that finitude is the greatest burden of human existence. However, when looked at more closely, it is also the prerequisite for its meaning, its seriousness and its dignity. The desire to overcome death will probably always accompany humanity; reconciling ourselves to finitude may be easier if we consider the actual consequences of biological immortality.

The Contradictions of Posthumanism

On the basis of what we have seen so far, the prospects for human biological self-improvement do not appear to be very favorable. Every conceivable optimization, seen in the light of day, very quickly raises conflicts between objectives which have been brought into a certain balance in the course of human evolution. One may imagine temporary shifts in these balances in favor of one side or the other but any permanent rebalancing must inevitably result in serious disadvantages. Even death, the "greatest of all evils," cannot be eliminated from our lives without bringing into question life's value and meaning.

In addition, any biotechnological perfection of human characteristics and abilities would promote the view of man as a machine that can be manipulated and optimized. Individual deficiencies and collective grievances would increasingly be interpreted as defects of human nature, which would have to be remedied technologically. Overhauling a defective product would replace personal development. Transhumanist utopias thus counteract the very efforts that have so far supported the idea of improving the human world—the efforts to achieve social, cultural, and moral progress based on individual and collective efforts, progress that cannot be achieved by technical reconstruction of the human being but only by self-education, self-development, and the common shaping of the lifeworld.

Yet, the idea of posthumanism itself is self-contradictory in a more fundamental sense. The desire to improve human nature still emanates from that nature; but its radical transformation would lead to a new, posthuman species, the "optimization" of which we no longer have any standards for. Transhumanists often proclaim that we could not even imagine the possibilities and forms of experience this new human being might have. According to Kurzweil (2005), it is no longer possible to make predictions about what happens after the revolutionary "singularity," i.e., the fusion of man and artificial intelligence predicted for 2045.[19] But then, this new man, *Homo optimus*, cannot be a meaningful goal for us—because we ourselves, *Homo sapiens*, would then no longer exist. The idea that we should transform into post-human beings is based on values, desires, or hopes that no longer fit these very beings, because they would have completely different values and desires from ours.[20] The creation of posthuman beings can then only be motivated by the paradoxical desire to eliminate *Homo sapiens* and make room for a new species. But the elimination of humans by humans is, as C. S. Lewis already stated, a paradoxical undertaking, since "the being who stood to gain and the being who has to be sacrificed are one and the same" (Lewis 1943/2009: 43).

A related consideration leads to the same result: if we pursue the freedom to radically redesign the human being to its logical conclusion, then it must also include the possibility of changing one's own wishes and will. After all, these desires too are only preferences randomly generated by evolution and we do not have to follow them. But then, we would no longer know what the good or the "best" should actually be that an optimization is to strive for. All enhancement and re-engineering of human nature is still based on a traditional set of values, but without its basis in present nature it would lose its meaning. The coordinate system within which we could judge something like progress would already have dissolved before any transformation took place. There would no longer be an

---

[19] Bostrom argues in similar terms: "... so we humans may lack the capacity to form a realistic intuitive understanding of what it would be like to be a radically enhanced human (a 'posthuman') and of the thoughts, concerns, aspirations, and social relations that such humans may have" (Bostrom 2005: 4-5).

[20] "When thinking the possibility of *posthumanly happy* beings, and their psychological properties, one must abstract from contingent features of the human psyche" (Bostrom 2008: 120).

Archimedean point, as it were, to which the posthuman world could be attached. Nietzsche's "revaluation of all values" is, seen in light, a paradoxical concept.

Transhumanist utopias are usually quite naive projections of human desires from the present time: intelligence, beauty, health, happiness, universal understanding, and philanthropy. But they are not consistently thought through to the end. Why should the new human not leave behind such ordinary aspirations? Why not choose Nietzsche's "blonde beast"[21] as the new model, or even a pure, amoral hedonism, as already propagated by the Marquis de Sade as a consequence of a radical materialistic world view? In principle, nothing would speak against it, because from the point of view of a possible posthuman species all moral concerns would only be the expression of a narrow-minded traditionalism. Finally, Dostoyevsky's parable of the "Grand Inquisitor" points to another possibility: why should we not relieve humanity of the burden of freedom to decide between good and evil? A socio-technological optimism of happiness that replaces individual freedom and entrusts the organization and distribution of well-being to selected engineering elites would pacify the present conflictual world and finally redeem self-destructive humanity from itself. The claim that this is in reality a dystopia can only be raised by those who still take the present nature of mankind as a yardstick—for the posthuman species it would possibly be the new paradise.

Mind Uploading or Transfer of Consciousness

Finally, let us turn to the last utopia of transhumanism: the idea of being able to "upload" human consciousness into digital systems and thus detach it from the biological organism. For this purpose, a technical process—admittedly fictitious as yet—is supposed to emulate the brain,[22] i.e., copy its neuronal structure in such a way that it becomes available for other systems:

> The basic idea is to take a particular brain, scan its structure in detail, and construct a software model of it that is so faithful to the original that, when run on appropriate hardware, it will behave in essentially the same way as the original brain. (Sandberg & Bostrom 2008: 7)

---

[21] With this term Nietzsche described the "higher races"' ferocious need to compensate for their cultural repression with cruelty against foreign peoples: "At the center of all these noble races we cannot fail to see the blond beast of prey, the magnificent *blond beast* avidly prowling round for spoil and victory; this hidden center needs to be released from time to time, the beast must out again, must return to the wild...." (Nietzsche 1994: 25)

[22] In computer technology, emulation (from Latin *aemulari* = to imitate) refers to a system that imitates another system in certain structures and performance, i.e., not only its output.

> If successful, the procedure would lead to a qualitative reproduction of the original mind, with memory and personality intact, onto a computer where it would now exist as software. (Bostrom 2009).

This "digital intelligence" (Bostrom 2009) would then inhabit a cyborg or android or live in virtual reality:

> Imagine yourself a virtual living being with senses, emotions, and a consciousness that makes our current human form seem a dim state of antiquated existence. Of being free, always free, of physical pain, able to repair any damage and with a downloaded mind that never dies. (Paul & Cox 1996: xv)

Frequently, reference is made to the allegedly foreseeable possibility of connecting the brain with microchips and feeding their signal patterns into the neural network. Brains could then be programmed with speech or other software, fed with new, undreamt-of reservoirs of knowledge and intelligence, connected directly to the internet or even to other brains; conversely, consciousness could gradually be outsourced to external structures (Kurzweil 1999: 90 ff.).

All this is of course far from being realized, and it is highly questionable whether the brain can be connected to electronic data storage devices at all. Up to now, brain-computer-interfaces are based only on very global derivations of brain activity by means of EEG or electrodes in the skull. The signal patterns are processed by computers and enable the test persons to steer a cursor on the screen or to operate a robotic arm simply by imagining movements. This is certainly a remarkable success, but the reverse direction, i.e., feeding and storing specific signal patterns in the brain, is to date completely impossible. The actual "programming" or fusion of the brain with digital systems seems far off in time, given the complexity of the neuronal system's internal networks and interactions. In the future, we will therefore continue to acquire foreign languages only by learning and practicing, not by ordering programs and "downloading" them into our brains.[23]

What about the possibility of a mind uploading? First of all, the structure of the brain consists of a network of over 100 billion neurons and several hundred trillion synapses with very different degrees of excitability, the so-called *connectome* (Seung 2012)—the thought of "scanning" or "copying" such a structure is adventurous enough. However, it becomes fantastic once one considers that not only the structure, but the entire, constantly changing activity of the system down to the transmitter distributions in the individual synapses

---

[23] The fact that the computeromorphic idea of a "download" into the brain contradicts all regularities of neuronal learning processes, which are based on repeated, embodied experiences with gradual adaptation of the synaptic structures, is rarely noted.

must be recorded—it is difficult to say what should still be "scanned" here. The firing of neurons may to a certain extent still be represented as digital information ("on/off" corresponds to 0/1). But this is only the tip of the iceberg; all processes below this level are analog molecular and atomic processes with ultimately quantum-physical fuzziness and in constant flux. One could just as well try to make an exact replica of a waterfall.[24]

But let us leave such objections aside and turn to the basic idea of mind uploading. We are obviously dealing with a peculiar amalgam of materialism and idealism: on the one hand, consciousness is reduced to neuronal processes in the brain and thus *materialized*; on the other hand, it is seen as the *pure form* of these processes, namely as patterns of information that can in principle be completely detached from the substrate and transferred to other carrier systems. This already mentioned functionalism is nothing more than an *idealism of information*. However, both assumptions, the materialistic and the idealistic, are equally blind to the living reality of the embodied person. In the following, I will first criticize the functionalist, then the neuro-reductionist prerequisite of the transfer of consciousness.

Critique of Functionalism

Mind uploading equates the mind with the totality of algorithmic processes in a complex system like the brain—i.e., with *software* that could basically run on any kind of sufficiently complex hardware or wetware, whether made of carbon, silicon, or synthetic polymers, of neurons and synapses or transistors and microchips. Consciousness is based on nothing more than the functional relationships between physical elements, not on the biology of the brain, and certainly not on its integration into the life process of the organism. Functional relationships, however, can be described as data or information structures and thus become available for digital reproduction, as neuroscientist Christof Koch, for example, puts it:

....

[24] Apart from that, all current scanning technologies such as electron microscopy are destructive, that means, the brain would die in the process of obtaining the connectome. Kurzweil does not go into this problem (cf. Kurzweil 1999: 90 ff., 195 ff.). Yet bold visions abound here as well, for example of scanning the connectome via nanorobotics ("endoneurobots" and "synaptobots"; Martin et al. 2019). The authors even hold out the prospect of thus creating brain/cloud interfaces, "allowing persons to obtain direct, instantaneous access to virtually any facet of cumulative human knowledge." Individuals could then engage in "fully immersive sensory experiences" and "might experience episodic segments of the lives of other willing participants [...] to, hopefully, encourage and inspire improved understanding and tolerance among all members of the human family" (Martin et al. 2019: 2). Shining prospects for humanity indeed!

> As long as we can reproduce the same kind of relevant relationships among all the relevant neurons in the brain, I think we will have recreated consciousness. (quoted in Kuhn 2016: 34)

The progress of artificial intelligence (AI) has given functionalism an enormous boost. The achievements of human intelligence do not appear to be tied to the brain, much less to consciousness. Of course, no artificial system has even the slightest idea of what it calculates or does. Obviously, the decisive characteristic of pain, feelings, or thoughts is lost in the functionalist conception—namely their being experienced. John Searle's classic "Chinese-Room" argument (previously mentioned on p. 21) still holds true: even an artificial system that can translate perfectly from Chinese or answer all Chinese questions appropriately, does not yet understand a word of Chinese. Meaning cannot be reduced to functional algorithms or syntax if there is no conscious subject that understands it.

However, the same applies to the feeling of joy, to the sense of warmth, or the taste of a Sancerre wine—no qualitative experience as such can be derived from data and information. And this is not only because of the irreducibility of "qualia," which are discussed in analytic philosophy of mind, but because all experience implies a basic *self-awareness or self-affection*. It is *for me* that I feel joy or warmth, perceive, or think. And this self-awareness is not based on reflection or higher-order monitoring of conscious states,[25] nor is it composed of intentional contents or information; rather, it is already present in primary experience, for instance comfortable, thoughtless dozing in the warm sun. It is a basal *sense of self* that forms the background to all of our experiences, a *feeling of being alive* that springs from our corporeality and which manifests itself in well-being or indisposition, specifically in hunger, thirst, pain, or pleasure. From a neurobiological point of view, this background experience requires not only neuronal activities in the brain but vital regulatory processes that involve the entire organism and are integrated in the brain stem and higher centers.[26]

There is nothing to suggest that this vital sense-of-self can be reproduced in digital algorithms. Let us take the example of pain: the unpleasurable quality, the "painful" element of pain, can be expressed neither digitally in "zeros" or "ones" nor physically in "negative charges." This is because the difference between zero and one or between plus and minus only seemingly expresses a difference in value: in fact, this difference is a mere convention. It does not imply anything "negative," anything painful. All digital signs or physical states are themselves

---

[25] This is in contrast to common higher-order or representational theories of consciousness (e.g., Carruthers 2005; Rosenthal 2005)—for a critique, see Zahavi (1999) and Thompson & Zahavi (2007).

[26] Cf. Panksepp (1998); Damasio (2010); Fuchs (2018: 138 ff.) and Chapter 4, this volume.

just pure positivity, facticity, and externality. In Sartre's terminology, they are only *in themselves*, not *for themselves*. There is nothing to suggest that a system which runs them could experience something like pain. The same applies for all striving, the condition of *being after something* and *being ahead of itself*, which distinguishes conscious life. Artificial systems only go through states; they are not ahead of themselves, and they do not care for anything at all. Take the example of a cruise missile or a drone: it is equipped with a goal-detecting program able to modify the flight of the missile according to a forward-mechanism that minimizes deviation from the goal. Of course, the missile does not "seek" or "discover" anything. Each correction serves only the internal setpoint regulation of the mechanism and happens purely momentarily, without referring in any way to a set goal. To this goal itself the mechanism remains blind and deaf. Only conscious beings move in the space of possible futures and experience their own movement *as purposeful*.

In other words, the core of consciousness, that which makes us feeling and wishing beings in the first place, cannot be grasped by information theory. It is inseparably bound to our corporeal, sensing, and thereby biological existence. What is pleasant and what is painful, what is good and what is bad, cannot be expressed by any algorithm. Digital information carries no values. And whatever data and information we take out of a human brain in order to copy it or transfer it into an artificial system of processors and circuits, the result would again only be "in itself," pure exteriority. An android or cyborg programmed with such data would in the best case be an insentient zombie. Immortality is generally conceived a little differently.

The idea of mind uploading is brought to complete absurdity if one thinks of the possibility of multiple copies. Imagine *per impossibile* a perfect digital replica of my brain, in whatever substrate, were actually to recreate my subjective experience. If this were the case, then the process could be repeated: I could be replicated twice, three times, or more.[27] In which of these clones would my original first-person experience then be located? Each replica would claim to be "me," would remember my life, would continue my identity; which of them would be my real successor?—But we do not want to pursue such abstruse thought games any further. It is already obvious that the idea of using the brain as a blueprint for immortality has nothing to do with reality and more to do with a naïve belief in the computer model of the mind. The human person is not a copyable sum of data, not a digital program but rather a living and

---

[27] "One obvious consequence of uploading is that many copies could be created of one uploaded mind" (Bostrom 2009: 207).

experiencing being. The idea of mind uploading does not even deserve the name of a utopia, because it is nothing more than a fairy tale.

Critique of Neuro-Reductionism

The second prerequisite of *mind uploading* would be the identification of brain and person. In a typical formulation:

> All that makes up a person, such as their mind, their consciousness, emotions, mem-
> ories, their identity, is physically saved in the structure and the processes of the brain.
> (Mathwig 2008: 80)

I will examine more closely this neuro-reductionist view, which is widespread today, elsewhere (see Chapter 4, this volume). Here it should be enough to refute one of its conclusions, which is crystallized in the thought experiment "brain in a vat": a brain, removed from the body by a fictive neuroscientist, could be kept alive in a nutrient solution and be fed appropriate information from a super-computer, such that it could produce the same experience, the same world, the same self as it allegedly does inside a living skull—we would not notice the dif-ference. This is because our experience, so runs the argument, is nothing other than a data structure in the brain itself, no matter where it is fed from.[28]

The thought experiment is intended to demonstrate that all self- and world-experience is produced exclusively in the brain, provided that it is supplied with the appropriate signals from the outside world. It is obvious, however, that the experiment only proves what it already presupposes: that experience is nothing but a data structure in the brain, no matter from where it is fed. But the brain is not a "Chinese Room," a closed system that only receives input and outputs output. Rather, it is continuously involved in feedback circuits of interaction with the body and the environment, and it is only through these interactions that conscious experience comes about.

Even a supercomputer could never simulate the homeostatic self-regulation of the organism, all the complex inter-weavings of neuronal, neuroendocrine, and humoral processes that involve the entire body and that underlie bodily self-awareness or the feeling of life (previously mentioned on pp. 22f.). These

---

[28] The neuro-philosopher Thomas Metzinger, for example, claims: "Ultimately, subjective ex-perience is a biological data format" (2009: 8) produced in the brain. "In principle, you could have this experience without eyes, and you could even have it as a disembodied brain in a vat. What makes you so sure you are not in a vat right now, while you're reading this book?" (Metzinger 2009: 21). John Searle is even of the opinion that we are already brains in the tank: "each of us is precisely a brain in a vat; the vat is a skull, and the 'messages' coming in are coming in by way of impacts on the nervous system" (Searle 1983: 230; see also Searle 2015: 77 f.).

processes are of biological and biochemical nature and cannot be represented in digital information. Nor could a computer simulate all the circular inter- actions between the brain, the perceiving and moving body and the environ- ment on which our experience and actions in the world are based. Looked at more closely, if the experiment were to succeed at all, no computerized vat and no moving robot would be sufficient for the experiment, but only an apparatus that would ultimately be nothing other than a living, sensory-motorically struc- tured body interacting with its environment.[29]

A disembodied brain is as much a functionalist fiction as mind uploading. The paradigm of embodiment is directed against such cerebro centrism: only as an organ of a living being can the brain also serve as a mediating organ for sub- jective experience. Consciousness is based on the continuous interaction be- tween brain, body, and environment. It is therefore not localizable, neither as an internal state in the skull nor as a data pattern in the brain—it is the overarching activity of a living being related to its environment. In other words, it is the human being who perceives, thinks, and acts, not the brain. And with every activity and experience the brain also changes, because it adapts to the higher- level functional circuits of perception, thinking and acting in order to mediate them better and better. This is what we call learning. However, it is not the brain that learns, but the human being who learns by means of the brain.

Transhumanism as Neo-Gnosticism

Let us turn once again to the basic idea of mind uploading. It is now even clearer that behind the transhumanistic visions there is a reductionist as well as a dual- istic conception of the human being: the phantasm of the fusion of mind and technology is an expression of a profound disregard, even contempt, for *life* and the *living body*. To free the spirit from the material body is the salvation which today's techno-utopians are offering us. Ultimately, this makes them the secular epigones of the Neo-Platonic and Gnostic teachings of the body as the "grave" or "dungeon of the soul."[30] The Gnostics of late antiquity saw the demiurge's (a kind of adversary god) unauthorized creation of the world and man as apostasy from the primordial divine light. In the earthly life, the purely spiritual soul of man, the *pneuma*, is connected with the dark matter of the body, which is for- eign to the soul, and thus becomes impure. But if the spirit can free itself from

---

[29] A more detailed refutation of the "brain-in-a-vat" argument is provided by Cosmelli and Thompson (2010).

[30] The characterization given by Plato (Gorgias 493a).

the body through moral purification and asceticism, then it can finally return to the *pleroma*, the sphere of light and deity.

Of course, from a transhumanist point of view, the pure spirit no longer consists of *pneuma*, but of data structures, of information. As a pure form, as a substrate-independent structure, it should in principle be separable from the body and transferable to another substrate. This functionalist idea sharply separates the *essence* of the mind from its *existence* and assigns priority to the essence. In contrast, the paradigm of embodiment stands for the phenomenological principle that existence precedes and underlies essence (Sartre 1946). Pure information lacks precisely the decisive factor of existence, namely *concrete individuality*. Information is freely convertible and arbitrarily transferable, but precisely this advantage is also its fatal flaw: it knows no individual perspective, no place from which the world could appear to a subject, because this place is nothing but the body. *Mind is alive*, and it could not survive in the dead circuits of a computer. And only our bodily being-in-the-world allows for the freedom that we have in the earthly world; the body is the medium of our life, of all our feeling, thinking, wanting, and acting.

The transhumanists have a different idea of our freedom: in their radical-dualistic, neo-gnostic view, the mind must be freed from the body, because we are only contingently trapped in mortal vehicles. In contrast, the idea of embodiment states that bodies are not dungeons and spirits are not angels, but both are indissolubly entangled with one another. Never will the mind be detached from the organic body and transferred into a computer. Our conscious experience, just like our personal identity, is based on physical existence—on the body which we are. This embodied and thus of course mortal individuation is the price we have to pay in order to experience the freedom and wonder of earthly existence.

Conclusion

Being a human of real flesh and blood begins to annoy us, as Dostoevsky said—we would rather "be born from an idea." This hostility towards the flesh today finds its expression in the functionalist-cybernetic paradigm: humans are information-processing machines, their consciousness and their personality exist as programs and algorithms. Progress consists, therefore, in updating the deficient body by means of information and biotechnologies and, finally, converting it into a synthetic product. This is because the corporeality of our existence is one of the last sites of resistance to digital progress.

> Our body of today is still the body of yesterday, the body of our parents, the body of our ancestors. [...] It is morphologically constant; morally spoken: unfree, unruly

and stubborn; seen from the perspective of the devices: conservative, unprogressive, antiquated, unrevisable, a dead weight in the rise of the devices. (Anders 1956/1994: 33; trans. T. F.).

Indeed, our embodiment sets an unassailable boundary for all functionalist utopias: a being of flesh and blood is not representable in algorithms. And insofar as our conscious experience is constitutionally embodied, it also cannot be simulated, copied, or transferred in the form of information. *All experience is a form of life*. Radical transhumanist utopias fail because of their complete misunderstanding of what it is that life is. They want to be "begotten by an idea," but the idealism of information is sterile. Mathematics begets no man.

Now, the fact that embodiment and aliveness are constitutive for our existence does not in itself make human nature sacrosanct. Just as we medically intervene in our body, we cannot categorically rule out inventions into our nature. But the idea of optimizing this nature inevitably encounters conflicts and contradictions, as we have seen. They come about with the attempt to shift the proportions of human capabilities and abilities as they have evolved in the course of evolution. These already represent meaningful compromises resulting from the conflicting demands on a complex being such as the human within a changing environment. Any transformation of human nature would therefore be associated with a high price, and it would have to be paid for with one's winnings.

Transhumanism ignores the fundamentally antinomic structure of our existence, which as embodied and earthly existence is necessarily bound up in polarities. Transhumanists want to get rid of these polarities and contradictions—as if there could be something like pure mind, pure happiness, knowledge without forgetting, and life without dying. But just as the mind cannot be separated from the body, so desire cannot be separated from suffering, freedom cannot be separated from limitation, and life cannot be separated from death. This inescapable dialectic of embodied existence can be illustrated with an image that is one of the most beautiful passages in Kant's otherwise mostly prosaic work:

> The light dove, in free flight cutting through the air the resistance of which it feels, could get the idea that it could do even better in airless space. (Kant 1781/1998, p. 129 A5/B8-9)

So, even doves need the resistance of the air for their movement, and to rise up against the gravity of the Earth they remain dependent on it. This is because movement is something physical, and as such it is subject to the dialectic of embodied existence: *What appears as resistance, aggravation or suffering is actually the precondition for success*. In the end, this applies to all areas of the conduct of life: we cannot keep one pole of existence and free ourselves from the other.

Even consciousness needs the materiality and heaviness of the body in order to exist.

Thus, it is also the specifically human abilities for self-reflection and freedom that must set necessary limits to optimization. The increased degrees of human freedom in comparison to the milieu- and instinct-dependence of animals have their own price. It consists in the fundamental instability and vulnerability of the human constitution as well as in the ambivalence of freedom. Freedom for good and freedom for evil are inseparable. In this respect, Rousseau's ambivalence towards human perfectibility was quite justified: granted, human development in the interaction of cultural and biological evolution has left behind all mere natural history. But it does *not* lead to perfection as a possible final goal, only to a balance between contradictory individual, social, and moral challenges that must be met again and again. The secular utopias of a self-transgression of mankind do not want to recognize this *conditio humana*. To reconcile oneself with the limits of human perfectibility is, of course, a task that is always being faced anew.

But, without anchoring our wishes and values in human nature, we would end up losing the frame of reference which lends meaning and significance to our lives. It is the bodily conditions of our existence that provide us with the elementary values: birth, hunger, thirst, pain, lust, and death. Life is better than non-life, food better than hunger, closeness better than rejection, love better than hate. Some things are good, others bad. We find the primary good because it is already inherent in our life, we do not choose it at will. Embodiment is therefore also the prerequisite for all moral judgements. Of course, the golden rule, Kant's moral law or the idea of the unconditional transcend our primary needs. But, without the physical-affective basis that our nature provides us with, all moral orientation would also lose its coordinate system. We would then no longer be able to say what the good actually is. Indeed, the very concept of optimization would be rendered meaningless. The abolition of man by man is an absurd undertaking.

It is therefore necessary to defend our corporeality as well as our bodily nature against its degradation and devaluation. Certainly, the fact of embodiment does not by itself pretend to tell us what the good, the Aristotelian fulfilled life looks like; it does, however, give us better indications of this than any technically induced happiness. The fact that we are all damaged, vulnerable and finite in one way or another actually makes us human. Let us therefore be content with the human condition and its inevitable imperfectability. It is perhaps not the best, but certainly not the worst thing that could happen to us.

References

Anders, G. 1994. *Die Antiquiertheit des Menschen.* Vol. 1: *Über die Seele im Zeitalter der zweiten industriellen Revolution.* München: Beck. (First published 1956.)

Arendt, H. 1976. *The Origins of Totalitarianism* Boston: Houghton Mifflin Harcourt. (First published 1951, New York: Schocken.)

Borges, J. L. 1962a. "Funes the memorious." In J. L. Borges: *Labyrinths.* Harmondsworth: Penguin (pp. 87–95).

Borges, J. L. 1962b. "The immortal." In J. L. Borges: *Labyrinths.* Harmondsworth: Penguin (pp. 135–149).

Bostrom, N. 2005. "Transhumanist values." *Journal of Philosophical Research* 30(Supplement): 3–14.

Bostrom, N. 2009. "The future of humanity." In J. K. B. Olsen, E. Selinger, S. Riis. (eds.) *New Waves in Philosophy of Technology.* Basingstoke: Palgrave McMillan (pp. 186–216).

Bostrom, N., R. Roache. 2007. "Ethical issues in human enhancement." In J. Ryberg, T. S. Petersen, C. Wolf (eds.) *New Waves in Applied Ethics.* Basingstoke: Palgrave-Macmillan (pp. 120–152).

Carruthers, P. 2005. *Consciousness: Essays from a Higher-Order Perspective.* Oxford: Oxford University Press.

Clark, A. 2003. *Natural-Born Cyborgs: Minds, Technologies, and the Future of Human Intelligence.* Oxford: Oxford University Press.

Condorcet, M. J. C. Marquis de. 1794/1822. *Esquisse d'un tableau historique des progrès de l'esprit humain.* (First published 1794) Paris: Masson et fils.

Cosmelli, D., E. Thompson. 2010. "Embodiment or envatment? Reflections on the bodily basis of consciousness." In J. Stewart, O. Gapenne, E. Di Paolo (eds.) *Enaction. Toward a New Paradigm for Cognitive Science.* Cambridge, MA: MIT Press (pp. 361–386).

Crockett, M. J., L. Clark, M. D. Hauser, T. W. Robbins. 2010. "Serotonin selectively influences moral judgment and behavior through effects on harm aversion." *Proceedings of the National Academy of Sciences* 107(40): 17433–17438.

Damasio, A. 2010. *Self comes to Mind. Constructing the Conscious Brain.* New York: Pantheon Books.

Dante Alighieri. 2007. *Divina Commedia.* Commento a cura di G. Fallani e S. Zennaro. Rome: Newton & Compton.

De Dreu, C. K., L. L. Greer, M. J. Handgraaf, S. Shalvi, G. A. Van Kleef, M. Baas, F. S. Ten Velden, E. Van Dijk, S. W. Feith. 2010. "The neuropeptide oxytocin regulates parochial altruism in intergroup conflict among humans." *Science* 328(5984): 1408–1411.

De Dreu, C. K., L. L. Greer, G. A. Van Kleef, S. Shalvi, M. J. Handgraaf. 2011. "Oxytocin promotes human ethnocentrism." *Proceedings of the National Academy of Sciences* 108(4): 1262–1266.

Ditzen, B., M. Schaer, B. Gabrieal, G. Bodenmann, U. Ehlert, M. Heinrichs. 2009. "Intranasal oxytocin increases positive communication and reduces cortisol levels during couple conflict." *Biological Psychiatry* 65(9): 728–731.

Dostoyevsky, F. 1993. *Notes from Underground.* Richard Pevear and Larissa Volokhonsky (trans.) London: Everyman's Library.

1

Fallon, S. J., M. E. van der Schaaf, N. Ter Huurne, R. Cools. 2017. "The neurocognitive cost of enhancing cognition with methylphenidate: Improved distractor resistance but impaired updating." *Journal of Cognitive Neuroscience* 29(4): 652–663.

Fuchs, T. 2018. *Ecology of the Brain: The Phenomenology and Biology of the Embodied Mind*. Oxford: Oxford University Press.

Griffiths, S. 2016. "Is Technology Causing Us to 'Evolve' into a New SPECIES? Expert Believes Super Humans Called Homo Optimus Will Talk to Machines and Be 'Digitally Immortal' by 2050" in *Daily Mail Online*. https://www.dailymail.co.uk/sciencetech/article-3423063/Is-technology-causing-evolve-new-SPECIES-Expert-believes-super-humans-called-Homo-optimus-talk-machines-digitally-immortal-2050.html, last accessed on 01.06.2021.

Gvirts, H. Z., N. Mayseless, A. Segev, D. Y. Lewis, K. Feffer, Y. Barnea, Y. Bloch, S. G. Shamay-Tsoory. 2017. "Novelty-seeking trait predicts the effect of methylphenidate on creativity." *Journal of Psychopharmacology* 31(5): 599–605.

Haraway, D. J. 1991."A cyborg manifesto: science, technology, and socialist-feminism in the late twentieth century," In D. J. Haraway: *Simians, Cyborgs and Women: The Reinvention of Nature*. New York: Routledge (pp. 149–181).

Hauskeller, M. 2011. "Is ageing bad for us?" *Ethics & Medicine: An International Journal of Bioethics* 27(1): 25–32.

Hauskeller, M. 2014. *Better Humans? Understanding the Enhancement Project*. London: Routledge.

Herder, J. G. 1967. "Ideen zur Philosophie der Geschichte der Menschheit. Erster und zweiter Teil." In *Sämtliche Werke*, B. Suphan (ed.). Bd. XIII. Hildesheim: Olms-Weidmann (First published 1784–1785.)

Hurlemann, R., A. Patin, O. A. Onur, M. X. Cohen, T. Baumgartner, S. Metzler, S., I. Dziobek, J. Gallinat, M. Wagner, W. Maier, K. M. Kendrick. 2010. "Oxytocin enhances amygdala-dependent, socially reinforced learning and emotional empathy in humans." *Journal of Neuroscience* 30(14): 4999–5007.

Huxley, A. 1932. *Brave New World*. London: Chatto & Windus.

James, W. 1950. *The Principles of Psychology*. Vol. 1. New York: Dover. (First published 1890.)

Jonas, H. 1992. The burden and blessing of mortality. *The Hastings Center Report* 22: 34–40.

Kant, I. 1781/1998. *Critique of Pure Reason*. Paul Guyer & Allen Wood (trans.) Cambridge: Cambridge University Press.

Krause, B., R. C. Kadosh. 2013. "Can transcranial electrical stimulation improve learning difficulties in atypical brain development? A future possibility for cognitive training." *Developmental Cognitive Neuroscience* 6: 176–194.

Kuhn, R. L. 2016. "Virtual immortality. Why the mind-body problem is still a problem." *Skeptic Magazine* 21(2): 26–34.

Kuo, M. F., M. A. Nitsche. 2012. "Effects of transcranial electrical stimulation on cognition." *Clinical EEG and Neuroscience* 43(3): 192–199.

Kurzweil, R. 1999. *The Age of Spiritual Machines*. New York: Penguin Press.

Kurzweil, R. 2005. *The Singularity Is Near: When Humans Transcend Biology*. New York: Penguin Press.

Lavazza, A., M. Reichlin. 2019. "Introduction: Moral enhancement." *Topoi* 38(1): 1–5.

Lee, D., T. H. Huang, A. De La Cruz, A. Callejas, C. Lois. 2017. Methods to investigate the structure and connectivity of the nervous system. *Fly* 11: 224–238.

Lewis, C. S. 2009. *The Abolition of Man.* New York: Harper (First published 1943.)

Lieberman, P. 2006. *Toward an Evolutionary Biology of Language.* Cambridge, MA: Harvard University Press.

Lieberman, P., S. Fecteau, H. Théoret, R. R. Garcia, F. Aboitiz, A. MacLarnon, … & P. Lieberman. 2007. "The evolution of human speech: Its anatomical and neural bases." *Current Anthropology* **48**: 39–66.

Löwith, K. 1953. *Weltgeschichte und Heilsgeschehen: Die theologischen Voraussetzungen der Geschichtsphilosophie.* Stuttgart: Kohlhammer.

Lupton, D. 2016. *The quantified self.* Hoboken, NJ: John Wiley & Sons.

Lurija, A. R. 2000. *Der Mann, dessen Welt in Scherben ging. Zwei neurologische Geschichten.* Reinbek/Hamburg: Rowohlt.

Martins, N. R., A. Angelica, K. Chakravarthy, Y. Svidinenko, F. J. Boehm, I. Opris, … & R. A. Freitas Jr. 2019. Human brain/cloud interface. *Frontiers in Neuroscience* 13: 112.

Marx, K. 1960. "Der achtzehnte Brumaire des Louis Bonaparte." In *Marx-Engels-Werke.* Institut für Marxismus-Leninismus beim ZK der SED (ed.). Vol. **8**. Berlin: Dietz. (First published 1852.)

Mathwig, K. 2008. "Mind uploading – neue substrate für den menschlichen geist?" In **Japanisch-Deutsches** Zentrum Berlin (ed.) *I. Deutsch-japanisch-koreanisches Stipendiatenseminar.* Bd. 57. Berlin: JDZB (pp. 79–83). www.jdzb.de/veroeffentlichungen/tagungsbaende/band-57, last accessed on 01.06.2021.

Metzinger, T. 2009. *The Ego Tunnel: The Science of the Mind and the Myth of the Self.* New York: Basic Books.

Moravec, H. 1988. *Mind Children: The Future of Robot and Human Intelligence.* Cambridge, MA: Harvard University Press.

Mohamed, A. D. 2014. "Reducing creativity with psychostimulants may debilitate mental health and well-being." *Journal of Creativity in Mental Health* 9(1): 146–163.

Montaigne, M. de. 1993. *The Essays: A Selection.* **M. A. Screech** (trans.) London: Penguin.

More, M. 1990. "Transhumanism: Towards a futurist philosophy." *Extropy* **6**: 6–12.

More, M. 2009. "Limitless life: The psychology of forever." In **C. Tandy (ed.)** *Death and Anti-Death.* Vol. 7. *Nine Hundred Years After St. Anselm.* Palo Alto: Rio University Press (pp. 239–274).

Nietzsche, F. 1980a. Also sprach Zarathustra. In **G. Colli, M. Montinari** (eds.) *Kritische Studienausgabe.* Bd. 4. Berlin: De Gruyter.

Nietzsche, F. 1980b. Nachgelassene Fragmente 1885-87. In **G. Colli, M. Montinari** (eds.) *Kritische Studienausgabe.* Bd. 12. Berlin: De Gruyter.

Nietzsche, F. 1994. *On the Genealogy of Morals.* **Carol Diethe** (trans.) Cambridge: Cambridge University Press.

Panksepp, J. 1998. *Affective Neuroscience: The Foundations of Human and Animal Emotions.* Oxford: Oxford University Press.

Pascal, B. 1995. *Pensées.* **A. J. Krailsheimer** (trans.) New York: Penguin Books.

Paul, G. S., E. D. Cox. 1996. *Beyond Humanity: CyberEvolution and Future Minds.* Rockland: Charles River Media.

Persson, I., J. Savulescu. 2012. *Unfit for the Future: The Need for Moral Enhancement.* Oxford: Oxford University Press.

Pico della Mirandola, G. 1942. "Of the dignity of man: Oration of Giovanni Pico Della Mirandola." *Journal of the History of Ideas* 3: 347–354. (First published 1486.)

Plato. 1997a. "Gorgias." In **John M. Cooper** (ed.) *Collected Works.* Cambridge: Hackett.

Price, J., with B. Davis. 2008. *The Woman Who Can't Forget.* New York: Free Press.

Rosenthal, D. M. 2005. *Consciousness and Mind.* Oxford: Clarendon Press.

Rousseau, J.-J. 2011. *Discourse on the Origin and Foundations of Inequality among Men.* H. Rosenblatt (trans.) New York: Bedford. (First published 1755.)

Sandberg, A., N. Bostrom. 2008. *Whole Brain Emulation: A Roadmap.* Technical Report #2008-3. Oxford: Future of Humanity Institute, Oxford University. www.fhi.ox.ac.uk/reports/2008-3.pdf, last accessed: 01.06.2021.

Sartre, J.-P. 1946. *L'existentialisme est un humanisme.* Paris: Editions Nagel.

Searle, J. 1983. *Intentionality: An Essay in the Philosophy of Mind.* Cambridge: Cambridge University Press.

Searle, J. 2015. *Seeing Things as They Are: A Theory of Perception.* Oxford: Oxford University Press.

Seung, S. 2012. *Connectome: How the Brain's Wiring Makes Who We Are.* New York: Houghton Mifflin Harcourt.

Sorgner, S. L. 2010. "Beyond humanism: Reflections on trans- and posthumanism." *Journal of Evolution and Technology* 21(2): 1–19.

Swartwood, M. O., J. N. Swartwood, J. Farrell. 2003. "Stimulant treatment of ADHD: Effects on creativity and flexibility in problem solving." *Creativity Research Journal* 15(4): 417–419.

Thomas Aquinas. 2008. *Summa Theologiae.* Latin-English edition, Vol. 1. Scotts Valley, CA: CreateSpace.

Thompson, E., D. Zahavi. 2007. Philosophical issues: Phenomenology. In P. D. Zelazo, M. Moscovitch, E. Thompson (eds.) *The Cambridge Handbook of Consciousness.* Cambridge: Cambridge University Press (pp. 67–87).

Trotsky, L. 2005. *Literature and Revolution.* R. Strunksy (trans.) London: Haymarket Boos. (First published 1924.)

Voegelin, E. 1939. *Die politischen Religionen.* Stockholm: Bermann-Fischer.

Voegelin, E. 1968. *Science, Politics and Gnosticism.* Washington DC: Regnery Publishing Inc.

Williams, B. 2010. "The Makropulos case: Reflections on the tedium of immortality." In D. Benatar (ed.) *Life, Death, and Meaning: Key Philosophical Readings on the Big Questions.* Plymouth: Rowman & Littlefield (pp. 345–362).

Zahavi, D. 1999. *Self-Awareness and Alterity. A Phenomenological Investigation.* Evanstone: Northwestern University Press.

Chapter 3

The Virtual Other: Empathy in the Age of Virtuality

Introduction

At the beginning of the twentieth century, E. M. Forster wrote *The Machine Stops*, a science fiction story that foresees the virtualization of reality (Forster 1989). Set in a far future, the human population has lost the ability to live on the surface of the Earth. Individuals are now forced to live in isolation from one another in subterranean honeycomb-shaped cells. A mythical, omnipotent machine supplies them with artificial air, nutritional pills, reading materials, televised entertainment, and every other amenity imaginable. It also provides them with visual telecommunication with others because people's bodies and senses have become too weak for them to leave their cells and engage in face-to-face communication. Generation by generation they have become so dependent on the machine that they eventually remain helpless when the first signs of dysfunction appear in its operating system. This continues until the day when the machine apocalyptically breaks down, leading to the extinction of humanity through the cold hard facts of life.

At the end of the twentieth century, the Wachowski brothers portrayed a similar dystopia in their film *The Matrix* (1999). Intelligent machines rule the Earth and harvest humans in huge plantations in order to use their bodies and minds as sources of energy. To this end, the humans' brains are fed a simulated reality called the "Matrix." Experienced reality is nothing more than an infinite series of digital symbols that flow over the screen at the beginning of the film. Virtuality and reality have become indistinguishable. Clearly *The Matrix* and similar films manifest a widespread apprehension that the digital world is becoming independent—a planetary artificial intelligence—and increasingly generating its own reality. Virtuality has become a central theme of the twenty-first century.

However, the question of what is illusion and what is reality is nothing new, having been a central philosophical topic throughout history. This line of questioning is specifically *human* because, in contrast to animals, we can doubt reality and imagine things that do not exist—i.e., we can think and act in terms

In Defense of the Human Being. Thomas Fuchs, Oxford University Press. © Suhrkamp Verlag 2021.
DOI: 10.1093/oso/9780192898197.003.0004

of "*as-if.*"[1] The *irrealis* mode in language—terms such as would, should, and could—is the verbal expression of our ability to fantasize, fictionalize, and virtualize. Until the twentieth century this ability remained first and foremost a key for opening up possible worlds, for drafting alternative projects, and for temporarily loosening the shackles of reality. Schiller posited that freedom exists in the space of play and artistic creation (i.e., in the space of "as-if"), rather than in the space of the work and daily toil. The position that human beings are fully human beings if and only if they are playing[2] could only be maintained on condition that the sphere of play remains in contraposition to the sphere of reality—that means, the exception rather than the rule. Today, however, virtuality permeates more and more of everyday life, invading our workplace, relationships, and free time. Visual media and digital communication dominate our lives to such an extent that we could barely cope with reality if they were to disappear. Thus, in a manner they have become a reality machine to which we are connected, much like the individuals in E. M. Forster's story.

As theoretical accompaniment to this development, constructivist philosophies and media theories prove themselves particularly fitting. The world of media images and telepresence suggests an epistemology in which the world itself is nothing more than a projection—be it a product of subjective perceptual schemata or a construct of data processing in the brain. Our sensory organization itself, so it is said, does not convey reality at all, but only generates biologically useful fictions suitable for survival, a "movie in the head," a "phenospace," or an "ego tunnel," as neurophilosopher Thomas Metzinger calls it:

> The contemporary enthusiasm for the penetration of humans into artificial virtual worlds overlooks the fact that we have always been in a *biologically* generated "phenospace": within a virtual reality generated by mental simulation. (Metzinger 1999: 243; trans. T. F.)

> Nature's virtual reality is conscious experience—a real-time world-model that can be viewed as a permanently running online simulation. (Metzinger 2009: 104)

It would then no longer be possible to distinguish between reality, fiction, and illusion; virtuality would be the norm, not the exception. In this "ego tunnel,"

---

[1] Of course, one can assume that at least in higher animals the search for food or prey implies an imagination of the desired object. However, this does not surpass the imagination of what is already known to the animal. By contrast, human imagination is able to construct *whole new objects* or *fantasy worlds*. To what extent higher animals, especially great apes, are capable of *pretense*, another kind of "as-if," is a matter of ongoing debate which I cannot discuss here; but see for example Mitchel (2002).

[2] "For, to speak out once for all, man only plays when he is in the fullest sense of the word a human being, and he is only fully a human being when he plays" (Schiller 1967: 107).

however, the only road to *other persons* is also a virtual one, namely, via internal simulation. The brain simulates the expressions and actions that occur in the other's body through the virtual activation of our own bodily states; it can then, in turn, project these quasi-experiences onto the other as if we were placed in her shoes. Here a convergence may be seen between neurophilosophical concepts and simulation theories of social cognition.[3] Empathy and social understanding are regarded as projections onto others of inner representations or models. To put it bluntly, one could say that the person who perceives the other is not actually interacting with him, but only with internal models or simulations of the other's actions.

Neuroconstructivism goes hand-in-hand with a societal development in which the difference between what is artificial and natural, between a picture and the original, between illusion and reality is gradually becoming blurred. To an increasing extent we live in what Sherry Turkle has called a "culture of simulation" (Turkle 2011: 4). Media as such present an ambiguous ontology: on the one hand, they *mediate* reality, based on an "as-if" of its representation; on the other hand, they tend to push themselves in-between the subject and the mediated reality, becoming independent, and finally present *themselves*. This applies not only to our cognitive but also our *emotional* participation in the mediated reality. Our affective relationships to others are increasingly based on mediation and virtuality.

Nevertheless, this development is dependent on our previously described capability for creating fictions, simulations, and the sphere of *as-ifs*. We will see that our emotional perception of the other, i.e., empathic intersubjectivity, often incorporates imaginative or fictional elements—indeed, that empathy may even disconnect from reality completely and turn toward fictions or illusions. One might say that we also connect empathetically with our own imaginations or projections. On the one hand, this results in the potential range of human empathy becoming nearly limitless; on the other hand, however, the further our empathy disconnects from direct, bodily experience, the more it tends to lose contact with the other as such. This implies the risk of the other becoming a mere image, a frequently misunderstood projection—a *virtual other*.

In what follows, I will investigate the particular relationship between empathy and virtuality. Can empathy be detached from the immediate, embodied contact with others and transferred to virtual relations? And if so, what changes does it undergo in this process? In order to answer these questions, I will distinguish between three modes of empathy: (1) *primary*, intercorporeal empathy;

---

[3] Cf. Gordon (1996); Gallese (2005); or Goldman (2006).

(2) *extended empathy* which is based on the imaginative representation of the other, and (3) *fictional empathy* directed to absent or fictitious persons. The last of these modes is characterized by an "as-if consciousness" which maintains the difference between fiction and reality despite the empathy that one feels for the fictitious person. On this conceptual basis I will then pose the question: what consequences may ensue for intersubjectivity and relationships in our society as a result of increasing virtualization of perception and communication? How is empathy transformed when it is increasingly directed to a virtual other?

Overall, the main goal of this chapter is to show that empathy is a complex, multi-level process that may well imply components of imagination, virtuality or the "as-if." As such, empathy not only connects quite easily with virtual or fictitious persons and situations, it is even stimulated by imagination and fictionality. However, this occurs at the price of an increasing danger of projections and illusions—a connection that is of particular importance in a culture of growing virtuality.

Empathy and Virtual Reality

The difficulty surrounding the challenging task of coming to an understanding of empathy reaches back to the concept's very genesis around the end of the nineteenth century. One finds the same difficulty in the current debate between competing theories: *Theory of Mind theory* (Baron-Cohen 1995), *simulation theory* (Goldman 2006, de Vignemont 2009), *theory of direct perception* (Zahavi 2001, 2011; Gallagher 2008), and *theory of bodily interaction or communication* (Fuchs & De Jaegher 2009; Froese & Fuchs 2012) equally claim to explain our everyday understanding of the feelings and intentions of others. This difficulty can certainly be attributed to the complexity of the phenomenon itself. Empathy develops in different modes and consists of various components. In the following, I will divide it into three modes, namely, primary, extended, and fictional empathy.[4]

Primary, Implicit, or Intercorporeal Empathy

Primary empathy is based on the personal encounter with the other, on intercorporeal interaction.[5] When we see someone burst into anger, we perceive

---

[4] Still another mode might be termed "iterated empathy" as put forth by Edith Stein (i.e., the perception of the empathy of another person connects back in a way to oneself, as when for example we experience shame because of the embarrassed expression of others). Her theory, however, is not discussed further here (see Stein 1989; Thompson 2001).

[5] Cf. on the concept of intercorporeality (*intercorporéité*) Merleau-Ponty (1960). It corresponds approximately to the stage of infant development until the end of the first year of life,

their feeling directly in their expression and behavior. This does not require an inner simulation of the anger that we first have to arouse in ourselves and then transfer to the other person; nor does it require a theory of human behavior that teaches us the meaning of a loud voice, clenched fists, or an angry expression. As Scheler (1973: 301 f.) already argued, we immediately perceive the joy in the smile of the other person, the suffering in his tears or the shame in his blushing, because we experience the other person primarily as a psycho-physical unity of expression. Of course, the resonance of our own body is also involved in this: the other person's expression of anger evokes in us feelings of tension, flinching, and a wish to withdraw, and these subliminal feelings feed into the perception of the angry person. Feelings become understandable in *expression* because this creates a bodily *impression*: you feel the other person with your own body, even if this feeling is not conscious as such, i.e., remains implicit (Schmitz 1989; Fuchs 2017a).

However, the impression that the other person makes on us, for its part, elicits an expression in us (e.g., a confused or anxious look), which is in turn perceived by the other and modifies his or her bodily state. As a result, both persons involved engage in a circular, bodily affective communication without even realizing it. Whenever two individuals encounter each other, their bodies thus enter into a communicative "choreography," to use Goffman's term: glances, gestures, and intended actions respond to the other's body, and their sensorimotor body schemes start to envelop each other. We may thus speak of an intercorporeal assimilation or *mutual incorporation* (Schmitz 2011; Fuchs & De Jaegher 2009; Froese & Fuchs 2012). In terms of the affective side of experience, this amounts to *inter-affectivity*, which means a continuous interaction and mutual modification of both partners' emotional states. This interplay provides an immediate feedback of one's emotions directed toward the other and thus diminishes the risk of merely projecting one's feelings onto them.

Extended, Explicit or Imaginative Empathy

In the previous section, I outlined the dynamics of intercorporeal communication which make up the foundation of primary empathy. Of course, the possibilities of empathic understanding are far from being exhausted by this primary mode. On the basis of our primary empathy, we also come to conjecture about the situation of the other and envision how it must be from his or her perspective: what could have made her so angry, so shocked, or so injured? Why was

which is also called "primary intersubjectivity" in developmental psychology (Trevarthen 1979): already at a few months of age, infants are capable of a differentiated perception of the emotional expressions of others.

she particularly vulnerable in the given situation? In doing so, we expand our understanding and deepen our empathy. But the possibility of putting oneself in the shoes of another goes further than the simple conjecturing about why *the other* feels the way she does: in fact, I imagine how *I* would feel and react if I were in the same situation. At this point we are certainly employing some form of simulation, which, however, I would prefer to term *perspective-taking* or *imaginative transposition*.

This component of empathy is without doubt very different from the first one discussed. To begin with, it entails an *explicit, cognitive operation*, namely, the conscious envisioning of the situation of the other, which often employs information about them that one could not infer directly from the situation at hand. Also, it involves an *imaginative operation*, i.e., a transposition into an "as-if" scenario (as if I were the other) which transcends the bodily or physical level. As a result, it seems necessary to differentiate between a primary, implicit, or bodily empathy and an expanded, explicit, or imaginative empathy. The latter already involves an element of "as-if" and thus of virtuality.[6]

Fictional Empathy

Let us now return to the connections between empathy and virtuality; a closer examination of these connections allows us to discover much more than just the notion of expanded empathy. Because empathy can also be extended toward fictive persons or non-personal agents, a phenomenon which I call *fictional empathy*. As causes and objects of this mode of empathy consider the following:

- inanimate or non-living objects like the geometric figures set in motion around each other in the experiment conducted by Heider and Simmel (1944), which then created the impression for the participants that a sort of friendship existed between a circle and a triangle;
- robots, avatars, or computers that demonstrate "as-if" intentionality (think, for example, about HAL, the onboard computer of the spaceship in Stanley

---

[6] In the wake of the discovery of "mirror neurons," the primary, intercorporeal form of empathy has often been conceived as a simulation too. According to this view, when we perceive others, neuronal mirror systems evoke bodily sensations that correspond to the perceived expression of the other, which are then projected onto the other (Gallese 2005; Gallese & Sinigaglia 2011). In fact, there is no "as-if" at all here, because one's own bodily sensations and tendencies of movement, which resonate in the encounter with the other, only implicitly enter into the perception of the other's expression. Moreover, many of the feelings perceived in others trigger not similar but contrasting bodily resonances, such as in the frightened or fearful reaction to an outburst of anger. The concept of simulation is therefore unsuitable for understanding primary empathy (Fuchs 2017a).

Kubrick's *2001: A Space Odyssey*, which develops more and more of a personal identity throughout the film and for which one feels some sort of empathy during the climax when it "dies");

- persons in films or in the theater;
- characters in novels, e.g., Oliver Twist or Anna Karenina;
- photos, portraits, letters, or other messages from persons who are real but not present.

Clearly, we are dealing with very different occasions and objects that can potentially awake fictional empathy:

- first, there are inanimate objects that stimulate our bodily resonance through their *qualities of expression* or movement patterns;[7]
- second, there are inanimate objects that suggest *purposefulness or intentionality* through their behavior (which is further increased due to the possibility of interacting with these objects, as in the case of computer games or in cyberspace);
- finally, there are persons who are only given to us via virtual means, e.g., in pictures, films, writings, or in our imagination; here we have to distinguish between real (non-present) persons and purely fictive ones.

Such catalysts of our empathy are almost always accompanied by an *as-if-consciousness* that can manifest itself in differing forms. One form is the peculiar consciousness of pictorial media: I perceive this picture *as* a picture or this film *as* a film, that means, I perceive its content *as if* it were real. There is what has been termed an "*iconic difference*" (Boehm 1978) between the picture as an object in the world and the world *within* the picture, and somehow we are aware of both modes of reality simultaneously.[8] Also, there is the consciousness we have when fantasizing: while imagining fantasy worlds we are still aware of our own imagination *as* imagination.

---

[7] This sort of stimulation is especially apparent when one observes how children interact with their surroundings. A child may call an empty balloon "that poor balloon," or may refer to a descending line as "sad," or experience a tea cup lying on its side as "tired" (cf. Werner 1959). Accordingly, children "breathe life" into their toys and experience them as possessing a sort of quasi-sentience.

[8] In his *Sophist*, Plato already tackled the problem that images display an ambiguous status between being and not-being: "Stranger: Then what we call an image is in reality really unreal. - Theaetetus: In what a strange complication of being and not-being we are involved!" (Plato: Sophist 240 b/c).

Another form of as-if consciousness can be found in symbolic or metaphorical comprehension (e.g., when a child pretends that a banana is a telephone), or also in role-playing games (e.g., when children pretend to be thieves or ship captains). Further, when we empathize with an actor on the stage, we do so at least with a latent awareness that he is only acting out his role. This becomes clear from the irritation or fright that would strike us if the actor were suddenly to "fall out of character" or suffer a real attack of weakness. In the case of the cinema film, the as-if consciousness is usually pushed into the background due to the viewer's deeper immersion in the action, but it remains latently present.[9] We suspend our knowledge of the fictionality of what we see; we give ourselves over to appearances while always keeping a balance—a sort of "double-entry bookkeeping."

Is there in fact a fundamental difference between real and fictional empathy? As regards primary or intercorporeal empathy one can indeed conceive of certain forms of fictionality that allow it to varying degrees—consider interaction with fictive actors in cyberspace or identification with movie characters that can achieve similar or even greater levels of emotional intensity than real encounters. We are indeed bodily present in virtual spaces; we feel our bodily resonance and emotional participation—even if there is no actual *intercorporeal* resonance. But secondary empathy or perspective-taking already contains, as mentioned previously, a component of virtuality, an as-if consciousness: here again, I don't really become the other when I put myself in his shoes, and I remain aware of this. This imaginative empathy can also become effective in novel or film characters. What then is the difference? Naturally, in states of fictional empathy we remain conscious of the fact that we are not actually engaged with a real other. Even the actor in a theater, although present, does not interact directly with us. Thus, it would be wrong to posit some sort of ontological illusion, as if we were actually confusing fiction and reality. Nevertheless, empathy remains possible, because by surrendering ourselves to appearances, we allow the as-if consciousness to fade into the background to such an extent that we may empathize with the fictitious figure no less (indeed even more) than with a real

---

[9] Woody Allen's film *The Purple Rose of Cairo* (1985) toys masterfully with our latent fictional consciousness. In the film, an obsessed female fan of a particular cinematic hero frequents a movie theater in which she follows the character's every move until one night he miraculously steps out of the screen and descends into the filled theater. The other actors in the film, which continues to play, get angry, and begin to break character while attempting futilely to get their fellow performer back into the movie. Allen emphasizes the play-within-a-play aspect of the unfolding fiction by giving the movie that the actor has stepped out of the same title ("Purple Rose of Cairo") as the one he has directed.

person. The so-called *paradox of fiction*—that is, the fact that we can feel deep empathy for a person like Anna Karenina who we know does not exist—is not based on an irrational attitude or even an illusion but on the ability of fictional consciousness to oscillate in the mode of "double bookkeeping" between the two views of the event.[10]

This split awareness is, however, a cognitively sophisticated achievement, an achievement stemming from early childhood (Fuchs 2013) that remains precarious and can also be lost—in which case the "as-if" gives way to an illusory reality. This is a classic motif in literature: Pygmalion's love for his self-created statue was already mentioned in the first chapter; infatuation obviously favors illusion and projection. We have also already met E. T. A. Hoffmann's Nathanael, who is enchanted by the mechanical puppet Olimpia, yet simultaneously, in a fit of madness, scolds and rejects his human fiancé, Clara, for being a lifeless automaton:

> He sat beside Olimpia, her hand in his own, and declared his love enthusiastically and passionately in words which neither of them understood, neither he nor Olimpia. And yet she perhaps did, for she sat with her eyes fixed unchangeably upon his, sighing repeatedly, "Ach! Ach! Ach!" Upon this Nathanael would answer, "Oh, you glorious heavenly lady!" [...] he never had such an exemplary listener. (Hoffmann 1885: 13 f.)

The exuberance of feeling annuls the as-if consciousness and empathy becomes a projection. The problem of the distinction between human beings and androids, which today is raised by science fiction films such as *Blade Runner* or *Her* (see previous p. 18), is already alluded to by Hoffmann in an ironic form when, in the wake of Nathaniel's sad fate, the young men of society demand that their beloved "... should do something more than merely listen – that she should frequently speak in such a way as to really show that her words presupposed as a condition some thinking and feeling" (Hoffmann 1885: 16). Being in love can undoubtedly blind one to the shortcomings of the loved one, but you certainly wouldn't want to overlook the fact that your beloved is a machine.

In psychopathology, psychosis is usually associated with a breakdown of the "as-if," which indicates the transition to delusion (Fuchs 2017b). In the clinical literature, numerous cases are described in which addictive computer gaming causes delusional empathy: at a certain point, the patients began to believe that their computers were alive and playing devious tricks on them (Podoll et al. 2000; Schmidt-Siegel et al. 2004; Mason et al. 2014). Thus, they became incapable of differentiating between the mediating *carrier-object* and the mediated

---

[10] On the *paradox of fiction* see Radford & Weston (1975); Lamarque (1981); and Carroll (2007).

reality as such; in other words, they lost the "iconic difference" which is constitutive for our consciousness of imagery (as previously illustrated). Of special significance is finally the phenomenon of "transitivism" in cases of schizophrenia (cf. Fuchs 2015). Here, perspective-taking in interpersonal encounters loses its "as-if" character and progresses into a conflation of one's self with the other, as can be seen from the following example:

> A young man was frequently confused in a conversation, being unable to distinguish between himself and his interlocutor. He tended to lose the sense of whose thoughts originated in whom, and felt 'as if' the interlocutor somehow 'invaded' him, an experience that shattered his identity and was intensely anxiety-provoking. When walking on the street, he scrupulously avoided glancing at his mirror image in the windowpanes of the shops, because he felt uncertain on which side he actually was. (Parnas 2003: 232)

In this example, it becomes quite clear that perspective-taking or imaginative transposition requires an as-if consciousness similar to that during the perception of one's mirror image. In order to interact with others, one must be able *to simultaneously alternate and differentiate* between one's own bodily perspective and the virtually imagined perspective of the other—i.e., one must be able to assert one's self in the face of the other. If this split awareness breaks down, then it may lead to a quasi-borderless empathy in which the subject loses itself in perceiving the other. The same applies, as in the case study, to seeing one's own mirror image. Thus psychopathology also shows us that the as-if consciousness remains fundamentally precarious; at the same time it makes clear how central for us is the ability to distinguish between being and appearance.

Interim Summary

Empathy has proven to be a complex phenomenon that consists, on the one hand of *implicit*, bodily components arising out of direct intercorporeality, and on the other hand, of *explicit*, cognitive, and virtual components, which are made possible by our consciousness of imagery and fantasies, i.e., due to different modes of as-if consciousness. Depending on the situation, these components will take on differing degrees of importance; we can also arrange them on the following scale according to increasing virtuality (Fig. 3.1).

This means: the more directly I am in bodily contact with an other and, as a result, the more integrated into a shared situation I am, the more active my

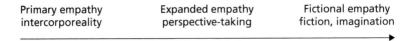

Fig. 3.1 Modalities of empathy

primary empathy becomes. And vice versa: the more that bodily communication diminishes, the more important the role of the virtual or imaginative
components of empathy become. On this spectrum, the degree of immersion—
i.e., the extent to which one enters into the virtual world and identifies with its
characters—is influenced by differing factors: literary texts enable us to directly
know the "inner life" of the characters through, e.g., inner monologues; films
heighten our empathy for the protagonists through, e.g., editing techniques,
close-up shots, the accompanying soundtrack, and so on. Finally, immersion
reaches a new level with virtual realities that offer the possibility of *interacting*
with virtual characters or avatars.

Of course, fictional empathy takes place within the realm of our imagination.
As a result, I remain to a certain extent within my own imaginative world, because many things can be imagined, and there is always the danger that I succumb to my projections.[11] The bodily presence of the other, however, possesses
its own resistance, because just as others appear for me in their body, so too do
they elude me. Bodily communication does not progress in a seamless fashion
(i.e., it does not signify a contagion or complete conflation), rather it entails a
subtle oscillation between resonance and dissonance that, in turn, helps drive
the process of interaction. In studies involving infants, Tronick (1998) was able
to show that affective communication between a mother and her child is precisely characterized by a shifting between "matches" and "mismatches," i.e.,
successful communicative mirroring but also disturbances in communication
followed by "repairs" of affect attunement. This is exactly the prerequisite for the
infant to experience itself as a separate being, delimited from its mother.

Even as adults we experience the other in every exchange as both opening
up to us through his face and expressions while simultaneously withdrawing
from us to a certain extent. Levinas (1978) even claimed that the possibility of
intersubjective experience depends on understanding the face of the other as
always having a moment of the foreign and the ineffable, thereby thwarting
my every attempt to reach a complete understanding—i.e., the other permanently transcends the world of my subjective impressions. Persons become real
for one another in so far as they acknowledge each other as beings to whom
"there is always more than meets the eye." They show themselves in their appearance and simultaneously remain beyond it. As we have seen, however,
this reality of the person can elude one's empathy if two conditions are met:
first, if the resistance in bodily communication is missing and the fictional

---

[11] This is why electronic communication favors (seemingly) intense relationships and the acceleration of emotional opening up, whereas real contact with the other "in the flesh" often
does not fulfill what the participants expected from each other.

component separates itself from the encounter with the other; second, if the as-if consciousness disappears and the difference between image and actuality, illusion and reality is lost. As a result, an illusory projection of the other replaces the face-to-face encounter.

Virtualization in the Present

Against this theoretical backdrop, let us now turn our attention to some current cultural tendencies toward virtualization, which were already mentioned in the introduction. A shared trait of the media and virtual worlds is a suspension of immediate bodily experience, a *disembodiment*, in which physical contact is minimized and the modalities of empathy lean in the direction of the fictional pole. To illustrate this phenomenon, I will characterize two aspects of disembodiment:

(a) phantomization, i.e., the dissolution of differences between image, illusion, and reality;

(b) disembodied or virtual communication.

Phantomization

As early as 1956, Günther Anders described "phantomization" *(Phantomisierung)* as the media-based simulation of direct reality: the surest way to obscure reality is to copy it constantly and everywhere, and indeed in such a manner that the facsimile-character of the copies themselves becomes so obscured that "the world disappears behind its copies" (Anders 1956/1994). As a result, reality, copies, and fiction become more and more difficult to tell apart. Forms take shape that lie somewhere between being and appearance which Anders named "phantoms," namely signs or images that appear in the guise of embodied things. Two decades later Baudrillard (1981, 2016) identified what he called the "simulacrum" as a media-based, simulated hyperreality which no longer allows one to differentiate between the original and the copy, between reality and imagination. Media sources (especially television) create a virtual contemporaneity with the whole world, i.e., a virtually shared world-moment. Originally, a constitutive element of imagery was the temporal differentiation between the image and that which it portrayed; it was always a *recreation* of its object. A simulation, however, goes hand in hand with the simultaneity of image and reality.

Instead of being just mediations, then, media sources come closer and closer to replacing reality itself. To still perceive an image *as an image*, i.e., to remain conscious of the "as-if" and thus to maintain the "iconic difference," is becoming increasingly difficult when one considers the image's evolution from a drawn or painted picture to photography, then to film, and finally to live broadcasting. In a quasi-hypnoidal state, the audience at some point gives up the effort of maintaining the difference between original and copy: the "as-if" breaks down. The illusion consists in allowing the copying of reality to be obscured and in forgetting that there also exists, for example, a real accident separate from the crash which the viewer sees in the televised car race. With long-running soap operas, reality shows, and interactive television, the medium itself tends to remove all differences between fiction and reality. The result of this development is what Anders named "*media idealism*": the world turns into a spectacle and the viewers become passive recipients of the images that media sources send them.[12]

On the other hand, it has often been suggested that the mass media themselves create reality by making events such as "9/11" and other terrorist attacks or rampages possible, or even causing them, in a certain sense, through their public portrayal. This further contributes to blurring the boundaries between image and reality. "9/11" consists more in its media images than in a real event; it is in a certain sense a single simulacrum.[13]

While the TV viewer remains a passive spectator of images, computing media integrate their users into sensorimotor interaction, regardless of whether it consists of virtual actions or verbal exchanges, and in the process enable new forms of immersion. As an interactive and communicative partner, the computer also becomes a potential object of empathy, which can even be ascribed personal attributes and quasi-intentions. The relationship to smartphones takes on almost erotic qualities, recognizable by the fascinated immersion in the screen and the

---

[12] "The world has now become mine, my idea (*Vorstellung*); indeed, it has transformed itself into an "idea for me," as soon as one is prepared to understand "idea" in two senses: not just in the sense suggested by Schopenhauer [Anders is referring here to Schopenhauer's *The World as Will and Representation* (Vorstellung)], but also in the theatrical sense [Vorstellung also means "performance"]. The idealistic element exists now in this *for me* ...." (Anders 1956/1994: 112).

[13] In this case, however, the ambivalent ontological status of a "media event" seems to have contributed to the mistrust of some viewer groups, which manifested itself in conspiracy theories of a staging of the attack. Similarly, one could assume that the current resentment toward the so-called "fake press" is a renewed awareness of the mediating character of media reality. However, this is not really a media-critical consciousness, because it is precisely the critics of a supposed manipulation who prefer to create their alternative reality from echo chambers of the Internet. All in all, we find a conspicuous tendency to blur the difference between reality and appearance, between truth and lie, to declare it unrecognizable or to abandon it altogether.

gentle stroking of the touch screen. The virtual reality of computer games and cyberspace then leads to the actual sensorimotor fusion of body and computer: no longer a passive spectator but transformed into an interactive agent, the user experiences a magical effect of his own activity, and the immersion reaches its ultimate degree. The illusion of bodily movement in digitally generated space promotes identification with avatars or other proxies, not to mention the empathic interaction with virtual persons. One could even speak of an "incorporation" of virtual space.

This would seem at first to contradict the thesis of "disembodiment" formulated above. However, it is in fact the almost perfect visual, tactile, and motoric coupling between user and computer that circumvents the experiences of resistance and foreignness that are characteristic of our normal bodily encounters with the world. This manifests itself not least in concepts such as "internet surfing," "browsing," or "skimming": they indicate the *minimization of resistance* in a medium that offers limitless possibilities for movement and, thus, an almost omnipotent self-experience. Consequently, the reality of the resistive body of flesh and blood is suppressed along with its multimodal sensations, its stirring emotions, and its need for food, drink, or sleep, in favor of a purely functional body coupled with a virtual media source, which in its functioning has become completely transparent. Its actual movement is reduced to a minimum. Thus, it is precisely the disembodied interaction with digital or visual media that may transition into highest degrees of immersion and thus illusion.

Disembodied Communication

Traditional televised media were the precursor to the replacement of real encounters through moments of pseudo-presence. In the meantime, however, virtual encounters are becoming increasingly a characteristic of everyday life *in toto*. Instead of interacting with embodied persons, we increasingly deal with apparent or quasi-subjects. We are served and questioned in detail by automated receptionists, we talk to Siri or Alexa; on the net we interact with social bots or other non-human actors, while we ourselves constantly leave electronic traces, images and data in virtual space, which in turn are exploited by anonymous artificial intelligence (AI) systems.

But even there where we communicate with actual others, this interaction is taking place in an increasingly disembodied form (Kang 2007). More and more areas of life are migrating to digital space, virtual communities are flourishing, as are filter bubbles and echo chambers. Even usually intimate encounters become *online dating* or *online psychotherapy*. On the net, however, the other person is "nowhere," she loses her physical presence and remains an intersection of various pieces of information that I acquire in the course of communicating with her. To what extent do self-stylization, constructs, fictions, and projections make up my picture of the other? The distinctions themselves seem to lose meaning. Undoubtedly, telecommunication accelerates and multiplies contacts, but without real encounters they lack the authenticity of bodily resonance. Instead, the cognitive elements of communication rule supreme.

This does not mean that virtual relationships entirely lack an affective cathexis—on the contrary: precisely because the non-sensuous means of communication leave so many blank spaces there remains even more room for the projection of feelings onto the other. However, what is really lacking is *inter-affectivity*, i.e., the direct feedback from the embodied contact, based on emotional cues and expressive gestures by which we perceive one another empathetically. Instead, the internet produces fictional or "phantom emotions" which are, as Eva Illouz has noted, directed not to the actual other but rather to oneself:

> Fictional emotions may have the same cognitive content as real emotions, but they are generated by involvement with aesthetic forms and are self-referential: that is, they refer back to the self, and are not part of an ongoing and dynamic interaction with another. In that sense, they are less negotiable than real-life emotions which may be the reason why they have a self-contained life of their own. (Illouz 2012: 210)

Such fictional emotions are triggered by linguistic signals from the other and may even become highly intense, though their actual object is absent. Nevertheless, since they seem to be directed to a real other who, after all, exists somewhere in the world, their fictional character is easily forgotten. Whereas the "as-if" is maintained in the case of one's empathy for Anna Karenina, it tends to elude one's awareness in disembodied relations to others, as for example in electronic dating procedures, where imagination and actual encounter are separated:

> [. . .] the style of imagination that is deployed in and by Internet dating sites must be understood in the context of a technology that dis-embodies and textualizes encounters, linguistic exchange being the means to produce psychological intimate knowledge. The intimacy that is produced is not experiential or centered on the body but rather derives from the production of psychological knowledge and modes of relating to each other. (Illouz 2012: 228)

Moreover, since electronic transmissions between opposite ends of the earth require nothing more than the click of a mouse, online interaction lacks the experience of foreignness and of growing intimacy. The space that would otherwise need to be crossed in bodily terms is removed; participants reach their addressee without a moment's delay. The novel space of virtual sociality is highly homogeneous: everybody seems to be equally near to me. The fine gradations between distance and intimacy are leveled out, and the nuances and retardations inherent in other social interactions tend to disappear. As a result, the virtual communication tends to produce a pseudo-intimacy, which those engaged would avoid if they were in direct contact. The other has become a mere projection surface, a product of my imagination, indeed, an object for my caprice. One push of a button and the virtual community disappears, as quickly as it was established: I wasn't actually ever *present* at all.

Summary and Conclusion

The increasing trend toward desensualization, as well as the proliferation of digital worlds of signs, of phantom imagery, and of illusory presences have all contributed to creating an artificial world, which, as philosopher Bernhard Waldenfels wrote, "inserts itself between seeing and the seen, saying and the said, between communicating and the communicated, between doing and deeds, between emotion and its expression" (Waldenfels 1995: 192; trans. T. F.). Recently, the Covid 19 pandemic with the worldwide lockdown measures has created an additional push for the digitalization and virtualization of communication, the effects of which are likely to permanently change our societies.

The culture of growing virtuality and simulation is connected with a disembodiment, a retreat from bodily and intercorporeal experience. Simultaneously, empathy tends to separate itself from these experiences and to shift into virtuality—into a space where we are confronted by hybrid forms of the other as a mixture of appearance, simulation and illusion, and where the medium and the mediated reality are increasingly confused. In the process, the prevailing modalities of empathy move from the intercorporeal pole toward the virtual and projective pole of the spectrum (cf. Fig. 3.1).

We still know too little about the long-term consequences of this development. Longitudinal studies have at least shown indications of a significant decline in empathic abilities since the turn of the century.[14] A probable cause might be the increase in virtual relationships and fictional empathy, combined with a reduction in interpersonal experience. It is true that virtual media create

---

[14] In a cross-temporal meta-analysis of 72 studies conducted between 1979 and 2009, Konrath et al. (2011) found that dispositional empathy in American college students showed a decline of over 40%, with the major drop occurring in the samples after 2000. The most pronounced decline was found in measures of *Empathic Concern* and *Perspective-Taking*. The authors point to virtual relationships and internet technology as one of the possible factors involved in this development: "With so much time spent interacting with others *online* rather than in reality, interpersonal dynamics such as empathy might certainly be altered. For example, perhaps it is easier to establish friends and relationships online, but these skills might not translate into smooth social relations in real life" (Konrath et al. 2011: p. 188)

extensive networks of weak connections that can be maintained and called up without costly investments. But the quantity of contacts in homogeneous virtual space is apparently increasingly replacing the quality of empathic relationships and deepened bonds in the bodily space of graded closeness and intimacy.

Of course, such developments cannot simply be halted, let alone reversed. Rather, we should follow them critically in order to constantly check whether we really want what we are currently doing. A culturally pessimistic lament is of little help in this regard. In view of the progress of digital media, more would be gained if we were to develop a refined awareness of the different qualities of social communication. It is precisely through the contrast with digital communication that we can recognize what bodily presence really means:[15]

- it does not merely consist of the alternating exchange of messages but also enables simultaneous communication, namely *active listening* with the signs of attention, questioning, or confirmation through glances or nods;[16]
- added to this is the empathic perception of expression, enabling *mutual bodily resonance*;
- the experience of the *direct encounter of the gaze*, in which the embodied intentionality of the person condenses;
- the possibility of *touching and being touched*;
- finally the *atmospheric feeling* of the presence of the other, which is based on the synaesthetic interaction of the senses. This shows itself not least in shared silence as one of the most intensive forms of physical co-presence, which is inaccessible to technically mediated communication (Böhme 2003: 141).

Key to our future dealings with virtual worlds will be that we do not abandon the ontological distinction between virtuality and reality. Anyone who flattens out the "as-if" of imagination and simulation, who declares the difference

---

At the same time, according to another meta-analysis, secure modes of attachment among college students decreased significantly between 1988 and 2011, while insecure modes of attachment increased (Konrath et al. 2014). It would certainly be premature to establish clear causalities here, but it can be said in any case that the new communication media have not increased the empathy and bonding abilities of American youth but have rather impaired them. In an even more comprehensive overview of the sociological study situation, Zarins & Konrath (2017) also come to the conclusion that, at least for the USA, a decrease in empathy and an increase in self-centeredness in recent decades has become undeniable.

[15] The already mentioned lockdowns during the Covid 19 pandemic have made this contrast more tangible than ever.

[16] Heinrich von Kleist described in unrivalled terms how such listening stimulates the thoughts and words of the other person (Kleist 1805/1964).

between image and original, appearance and reality, to be insignificant, will also contribute to populist manipulation, fake news, and ultimately to a disintegration of the common public sphere. Postmodern constructivism belongs to such tendencies: it gains its apparent plausibility from a cultural and media development in which the aforementioned distinctions, superficially seen, become blurred. This makes critical differentiation all the more necessary today.

Thus, there are good reasons for denying the thesis that the world is nothing more than a mental construct or a movie inside our heads. Perceptions are not representations or ideas, and even our ideas are constantly being either confirmed or proven false by the world. To maintain such a corrective relationship, however, two conditions are required: first, that one actively deals with the world and, second, that one experiences concrete encounters with others. Both conditions act as checks and balances for our preconceptions, ideas, and illusions. In our interaction with the world, the corrections take place via direct reaction, success, and failure; in our direct encounters with others, via resistance, the foreignness of the other, and the oscillation of perspectives that every encounter sets in motion.

A final criterion of reality is that it is entails surprises or unexpected events which jolt us and which we can never predict. That which is real reveals itself through an otherness, unpredictability, and resistance that must be overcome again and again.[17] Conversely, reality disappears to the extent that it becomes "compliant," i.e., frictionless, saturating the senses, and circumventing attentive, critical perception. Moving and interactive images are especially well suited for dominating one's senses, capturing one's gaze, and connecting directly to one's imagination. It is not for nothing that throughout humanity's cultural development images have been thought to possess mythical powers, which has often lead to their becoming taboo or prohibited in the attempt to curtail their magical and transformative force. We live, however, in a society that is free of any such prohibition—and where the flood of images is accordingly greater than at any other time in history. For a long time, the sense of sight has become the dominant sense of our ocularcentric society. But sight knows no resistance, and it is the most easily deceived of all the senses. If we desire direct contact with concrete reality, then we must learn to stem the tide of images and to reconnect our sensuous experiences with our embodied presence.

Crucial in this context is the question of the reality of the other. If all real life consists in encounters, as Martin Buber says (Buber 1958: 25), then the

---

[17] One could argue that components of surprise and resistance are also part of virtual games. However, here they belong to the preset framework of the game and, as such, are expected by the player.

manner in which we encounter one another will decide the extent to which we are in tune with reality at all. The other is the only being who transcends the bare world as given "for me," beyond media-based idealism or the neuro-constructivist inner space from which we can ostensibly never escape. Only the other frees me from the cage of my imaginings and projections in which I only ever encounter myself. The ethical claim that comes from the other is ultimately wrapped up in his physical presence: in his gaze, in the sound of his voice, in his face. And only when others become real for us in this manner can we become real for ourselves. Today, our relationships come increasingly to be mediated, even produced, by images. But no one encounters us through a smartphone. The virtual presence of the other cannot replace intercorporeality.

References

Anders, G. 1994. *Die Antiquiertheit des Menschen*, Bd. I.: *Über die Seele im Zeitalter der zweiten industriellen Revolution*. München: Beck. (First published 1956.)

Baron-Cohen, S. 1995. *Mindblindness: An Essay on Autism and Theory of Mind*. Cambridge, MA: MIT Press.

Baudrillard, J. 1981. Requiem for the media. In *For a Critique of the Political Economy of the Sign*. C. Levin (trans.) Saint Louis/Missouri: Telos Press (pp. 164–184).

Baudrillard, J. 2016. *Symbolic Exchange and Death*. I. H. Grant (trans.). Los Angeles, London: Sage.

Boehm, G. 1978. "Zu einer Hermeneutik des Bildes." In H.-G. Gadamer, G. Boehm (eds.) *Die Hermeneutik und die Wissenschaften*. Frankfurt/M.: Suhrkamp (pp. 444–447).

Böhme, G. 2003. *Leibsein als Aufgabe: Leibphilosophie in pragmatischer Hinsicht*. Kusterdingen: Die Graue Edition.

Buber, M. 1984. *Das Dialogische Prinzip*. Heidelberg: Lambert Schneider.

Carroll, N. 2007. *The Philosophy of Motion Pictures*. London: Blackwell.

de Vignemont, F. 2009. "Drawing the boundary between low-level and high-level mindreading." *Philosophical Studies* 144: 457–466.

Forster, E. M. 1989. "The Machine Stops." In E. M. Forster (ed.) *Collected Short Stories*. London: Penguin Books. (First published 1909.)

Froese, T., T. Fuchs. 2012. "The extended body: A case study in the neurophenomenology of social interaction." *Phenomenology and the Cognitive Sciences* 11: 205–236.

Fuchs, T. 2013. "The phenomenology and development of social perspectives." *Phenomenology and the Cognitive Sciences* 12: 655–683.

Fuchs, T. 2015. "Pathologies of intersubjectivity in autism and schizophrenia." *Journal of Consciousness Studies* 22: 191–214.

Fuchs, T. 2017a. "Intercorporeality and interaffectivity." In C. Meyer, J. Streeck, S. Jordan (eds.) *Intercorporeality: Emerging Socialities in Interaction*. Oxford: Oxford University Press (pp. 3–24).

Fuchs, T. 2017b. "The 'as if' function and its loss in schizophrenia." In M. Summa, T. Fuchs, L. Vanzago (eds.) *Imagination and Social Perspectives. Approaches from Phenomenology and Psychopathology*. New York, London: Routledge (pp. 83–98).

Fuchs, T., H. De Jaegher. 2009. "Enactive intersubjectivity: Participatory sense-making and mutual incorporation." *Phenomenology and the Cognitive Sciences* 8: 465–486.

Gallagher, S. 2008. "Direct perception in the intersubjective context." *Consciousness and Cognition* 17: 535–543.

Gallese, V. 2005. "Embodied simulation: From neurons to phenomenal experience." *Phenomenology and the Cognitive Sciences* 4: 23–48.

Gallese, V., C. Sinigaglia. 2011. "What is so special about embodied simulation?" *Trends in Cognitive Sciences* 15: 512–519.

Goldman, A. 2006. *Simulating Minds. The Philosophy, Psychology, and Neuroscience of Mindreading*. Oxford: Oxford University Press.

Heider, F., M. Simmel. 1944. "An experimental study of apparent behavior." *American Journal of Psychology* 57: 243–259.

Hoffmann, E. T. A. 1885. *The Sand-Man*. J. Y. Bealby (trans.) New York: Charles Scribner's Sons (http://faculty.washington.edu/jdwest/russ430/sandman.pdf).

Illouz, E. 2012. *Why Love Hurts. A Sociological Explanation*. Cambridge: Polity Press.

Kang, S. 2007. "Disembodiment in online social interaction: Impact of online chat on social support and psychosocial well-being." *CyberPsychology & Behavior* 10(3): 475–477.

Kleist, H. 1964. "Über die allmähliche Verfertigung der Gedanken beim Reden." In *Sämtliche Werke*. P. Stapf (ed.). Berlin, Darmstadt, Wien: Wissenschaftliche Buchgesellschaft (pp. 1032–1037). (Erstausgabe 1805.)

Konrath, S. H., E. H. O'Brien, C. Hsing. 2011. "Changes in dispositional empathy in American college students over time: A meta-analysis." *Personality and Social Psychology Review* 15: 180–198.

Konrath, S. H., W. J. Chopik, C. Hsing, E. H. O'Brien. 2014. "Changes in adult attachment styles in American college students over time: A meta-analysis." *Personality and Social Psychology Review* 18: 326–348.

Lamarque, P. 1981. "How can we fear and pity fictions?" *British Journal of Aesthetics* 21: 291–304.

Levinas, E. 1978. *Otherwise than Being or Beyond Essence*. A. Lingis (trans.). Dordrecht: Kluwer Academic Publishers.

Mason, O. J., C. Stevenson, F. Freedman. 2014. "Ever-Present Threats from Information Technology: The Cyber-Paranoia and Fear Scale." *Frontiers in Psychology* 5: 1298.

Merleau-Ponty, M. 1960. "Le philosophe et son ombre." In M. Merleau-Ponty (ed.) *Signes*. Paris: Éditions Gallimard (pp. 158–179).

Metzinger, T. 1999. *Subjekt und Selbstmodell*. Paderborn: Mentis.

Metzinger, T. 2009. *The Ego Tunnel: The Science of the Mind and the Myth of the Self*. New York: Basic Books.

Parnas, J. 2003. "Self and schizophrenia: A phenomenological perspective." In T. Kircher, A. David (eds.) *The Self in Neuroscience and Psychiatry*. Cambridge: Cambridge University Press (pp. 217–241).

Plato. 1997. "Sophist." N. P. White (trans.). In John M. Cooper (ed.) *Collected Works*. Cambridge: Hackett (pp. 235–293).

Podoll, K., E. Habermeyer, B. Nöller, H. Ebel, H. Sass. 2000. "Internet als Wahnthema bei paranoider Schizophrenie." *Nervenarzt* 71: 912–914.

Radford, C., M. Weston. 1975. "How can we be moved by the fate of Anna Karenina?" *Proceedings of the Aristotelian Society* (49) (Supplement): 67–93.

Scheler, M. 1973. "Wesen und Formen der Sympathie." In M. Scheler and M. S. Frings (eds.) *Gesammelte Werke*, Bd. 9. Bern, München: Francke (Erstausgabe 1923.)

Schiller, F. 1967. *On the Aesthetic Education of Man: In a Series of Letters*. E. M. Wilkinson, L. A. Willoughby (trans.). Oxford: Clarendon Press.

Schmidt-Siegel, B., T. Stompe, G. Ortwein-Swoboda. 2004. "Being a webcam." *Psychopathology* 37: 84–85.

Schmitz, H. 1989. "Über leibliche Kommunikation." In H. Schmitz, *Leib und Gefühl. Materialien zu einer Philosophischen Therapeutik*. Paderborn: Junfermann (pp. 175–218).

Schmitz, H. 2011. *Der Leib*. Berlin: De Gruyter.

Stein, E. 1989. *On the Problem of Empathy*. W. Stein, Trans. Washington, D.C.: ICS Publications.

Thompson, E. 2001. "Empathy and consciousness." *Journal of Consciousness Studies* 8: 1–32.

Trevarthen, C. 1979. "Communication and cooperation in early infancy: A description of primary intersubjectivity." In M. Bullowa (ed.) *Before Speech. The Beginning of Interpersonal Communication*. Cambridge: Cambridge University Press (pp. 321–347).

Tronick, E. Z. 1998. "Dyadically expanded states of consciousness and the process of therapeutic change." *Infant Mental Health Journal* 19: 290–299.

Turkle, S. 2011. *Alone Together. Why We Expect More from Technology and Less from Each Other*. New York: Basic Books.

Waldenfels, B. 1995. "Ein menschlicher Traum für Wachende." In H. Lenk, H. Poser (eds.) *Neue Realität: Herausforderung der Philosophie*. Berlin: Akademie Verlag (pp. 190–204).

Werner, H. 1959. *Einführung in die Entwicklungspsychologie*. München: Barth.

Zahavi, D. 2001. "Beyond empathy. Phenomenological approaches to intersubjectivity." *Journal of Consciousness Studies* 8: 151–167.

Zahavi, D. 2011. "Empathy and direct social perception: A phenomenological proposal." *Review of Philosophy and Psychology* 2: 541–558.

Zarins, S., S. Konrath. 2017. "Changes over time in compassion-related variables in the United States." In E. M. Seppälä, E. Simon-Thomas, S. L. Brown, M. C. Worline, C. D. Cameron, J. R. Doty (eds.) *The Oxford Handbook of Compassion Science*. Oxford: Oxford University Press (pp. 331–352).

B

Brain, Person, and Reality

Chapter 4

Person and Brain: Against Cerebrocentrism

Introduction

Do we find what constitutes a person in the brain? Do a person's perceptions, thoughts, feelings, and desires show up in the brightly colored computer images of brain processes? Are the love, happiness, or guilt that a person feels ultimately neural states? Neurobiology, at least in its currently dominant interpretation, claims exactly this. A view into the skull becomes, for the neurobiologist, a view into the innermost part of the person, into his or her wishes and fears, happiness and suffering:

> Our thoughts and our dreams, our memories and experiences all arise from this strange neural material. Who we are is found within the intricate firing patterns of electrochemical impulses. (Eagleman 2015: 5)

For neurobiology, the brain becomes the new subject, the thinker of our thoughts and doer of our actions; subjectivity itself is only a useful illusion:

> Ultimately, subjective experience is a biological data format, a highly specific mode of presenting information about the world by letting it appear as if it were an Ego's knowledge. But no such things as selves exist in the world. (Metzinger 2009: 23)

Another popular illustration of this view is the thought experiment introduced by Hilary Putnam (1981) into the brain-mind debate, namely the "*brain in a vat*": if we were only brains in a nutrient solution, suitably stimulated by a computer, Putnam says, we would not notice the fact. The brain would hallucinate a subject and a world that resembled our experienced world completely— a perfect illusion like the computer-generated world of the film *The Matrix*. Metzinger also considers ordinary visual perception to be a kind of online hallucination, a technicolor film produced by the brain: "In principle, you could have this experience without eyes, and you could even have it as a disembodied brain in a vat" (Metzinger 2009: 21). The thought experiment of a *brain transplant* seems to lead to a comparable result. If the brain of person A were transplanted into the body of person B, then it would not be B who would receive a new brain, but A a new body—where the brain is, there must also be the person. "This simple fact," says neuroscientist Gazzaniga, "makes it clear that you are

In Defense of the Human Being. Thomas Fuchs, Oxford University Press. © Suhrkamp Verlag 2021.
DOI: 10.1093/oso/9780192898197.003.0005

your brain. The neurons interconnecting in its vast network, discharging in certain patterns modulated by certain chemicals, controlled by thousands of feedback networks—that is you" (Gazzaniga 2005: 31). Of course, this is anything but a fact. Yet the brain seems to be the only part of the body that we need to have in order to be ourselves; the rest is interchangeable. Persons are cerebral subjects, and images of the brain are the modern icons of the person.

Another development contributes to the identification of person and brain, namely the rationalistic conception of personal identity, which goes back to John Locke (1689). According to him, this identity is based solely on conscious memory and self-consciousness, not on physical existence.[1] I remain myself as long as I can remember and ascribe my former states to myself; otherwise my identity would be destroyed. This psychologization of the person meant a radical departure from the Aristotelian position according to which persons were basically living beings embodied in a physical body. Since the brain was now increasingly regarded as the seat of memory and consciousness, Locke's reinterpretation also encouraged the equation of person and brain (Vidal 2011).

All these views of personhood have one thing in common: they are based on the ultimately dualistic premise that there is only consciousness and brain, the mental and the physical. The *living being*, the living organism as the underlying unit, however, no longer appears. Conscious activities are not regarded as functions of an organism but are equated with brain processes. In this view, the body remains a mere carrier apparatus for the brain, in which the incorporeal inner world of consciousness and thus also the person is created. In what follows, this neuro-reductionist concept of personhood will be subjected to critique.[2] The counter-thesis, which I then elaborate, will be this: the brain is only an *organ* of the person, not the seat of the person. In other words: *personhood means embodied subjectivity*.

---

[1] In his *Essay Concerning Human Understanding* (1689), Locke defines the person as "a thinking intelligent being, that has reason and reflection, and can consider itself as itself, the same thinking thing in different times and places" (Locke 1689/1997: 302). Personal identity consequently consists in the continuity of memory and self-consciousness: "as far as this consciousness can be extended backwards to any past action or thought, so far reaches the identity of that *person*" (Locke 1689/1997: 302).

[2] For similar approaches to a "critical neuroscience," see in particular Slaby (2010); Choudhuri & Slaby (2012).

Critique of the Cerebral Subject

In the critique it must first be shown that subjectivity is not to be found inside the body, i.e., it cannot be identified with the brain. It is even more true for the concept of the person that it eludes a neurobiological comprehension.

Subjectivity and Intentionality

Is the brain the locus of subjectivity and consciousness? Let's start with Leibniz's well-known comparison from his *Monadology*:

> And supposing there were a machine, so constructed as to think, feel, and have perception, it might be conceived as increased in size, while keeping the same proportions, so that one might go into it as into a mill. That being so, we should, on examining its interior, find only parts which work one upon another, and never anything by which to explain a perception. (Leibniz 1714/2009: 17)

This still applies today. Whoever examines the brain of a human being finds nerve cells and electrochemical processes, but never the person's fear or pain, their sensations or thoughts. Neither neurons, nor brain centers, nor brains as a whole are subjects of an experience. The visual cortex is undoubtedly necessary for seeing, but it itself sees nothing at all, because seeing, perceiving, and feeling are *activities of living beings*. Dogs, cats, and humans see something; it is not their brains that see. Anyone who tries to find seeing *within* a living being has already overlooked it by looking too closely.

So, when brain researchers claim that consciousness is undoubtedly located in the brain, they are subject to a category mistake. *People* are conscious, not brains. The fact that we cannot see "consciousness" but only conscious people does not mean that experience can be found in a hidden place inside. Consciousness is not at all a localizable object to which one could point like we can point to a stone or an apple, but a relationship between subject and world. It is a perception of …, speaking with …, desiring something, etc., that is, a directed process that *opens up a world*. This intentional relationship of subject and world cannot be reified or locked up in the skull. "*Where* then is the consciousness, the perception, the thinking?" Leibniz' comparison already shows: the question itself is wrongly posed.

A second objection: is subjective experience at all objectifiable? Can it be described in objective, e.g., neurobiological terms?—Thomas Nagel has shown that every subjective experience is tied to a centered perspective that cannot be reconstructed in an objective, physical description (Nagel 1974). How does it feel to have exactly *this* pain, to experience *this* fear? Can the fact that I am feeling pain be described from a third-person perspective too, namely as a certain neuronal activity pattern in my brain? No, because even the reformulation

"Thomas Fuchs is now in pain" no longer expresses the fact that it is *my* pain and that it is *I* who suffers from it.[3] Even if this statement were to be reliably true in all cases from the third-person perspective (for example, on the basis of simultaneous observation of my brain processes), it would still lack the decisive characteristic of subjectivity, namely that *I myself* am precisely the Thomas Fuchs to whom the statement refers. This would be even more true for an exact description of all the physical processes in my brain—nowhere in such descriptions could one find the "mineness" or the "painfulness" of my pain. Between the two ways of talking about pain lies a categorical gap: the reality of my pain is of a *fundamentally different kind* than the reality of objective physical facts—and in a certain sense it is even more "real" than these.[4]

Embodiment

The objections against neuro-reductionism mentioned so far are based on the irreducible intentionality and subjectivity of personal consciousness. But the scope of the concept of person is not yet exhausted. The fact that a person's life conduct cannot be identified with brain processes becomes even more apparent when we look beyond pure consciousness to the living reality of the person. This clearly rests upon the person's *embodiment*, not only in the sense that consciousness presupposes a functional body, but also in the sense that persons realize and represent themselves in their body, and that we can *identify* persons with their physical appearance each time we encounter them.

Most of our activities are tied to the medium of the body. In order to be able to feel, hear, see or speak, we obviously need not only a brain but also a feeling, hearing, seeing, and speaking body. It is not that we thereby use the body as a mere external instrument. When I dance a waltz, I do not set my limbs in motion from the outside but *I myself am the one* who dances, by swinging to the rhythm of the music and executing my movements kinesthetically. An experienced dancer, actor, or pianist is therefore unlikely to get the idea of identifying himself with his head or brain. My body possesses its own "operative intentionality"

---

[3] This has been shown in detail by Hermann Schmitz, whose fundamental analysis of subjective facts I follow here: "A fact [...] is *subjective* if at most *one person*, and only in his own name, can declare it, while the others can speak about it with clear identification, but can never ever declare what is meant" (Schmitz 1995: 6).

[4] Cf. Schmitz once more: "Subjective facts are, so to speak, actual to a greater extent than objective facts; they have the vividness of what is full-blooded and urgently real, whereas the merely objective world, constituted by objective facts alone, is something like a chemical preparation, diluted and made ready for narratives in the grammatical third person". (Schmitz 1995: 7)

(Merleau-Ponty 1962), its movements are meaningful, purposeful, and adapted to the environment without me having to control them from the outside.

Of course, this also requires corresponding neural dispositions, namely patterns of movement sequences in the motor cortex, the cerebellum, and the basal ganglia. But even these do not "control" or "determine" my limbs as if they were mere executing organs. Rather, the neuronal functions themselves are embedded in the constant interaction of: (1) bodily movement, (2) reaction and resistance of the environment, and (3) kinesthetic, tactile, and visual perception. The body, with its senses and limbs, is the actual "player on the field," while the brain acts as a mediator that connects and continuously modifies these feedback interactions (Fuchs 2011). I dance and move as a living, bodily being, *mediated* by my brain—but I do not set my limbs in motion from the brain like a homunculus.

My embodiment therefore fundamentally shapes my personal way of being in the world too. To find myself as *this* body, to have *this* shape and constitution, to be a child or adult, man or woman, small or large, healthy or handicapped, is the starting point of all self- and world-experience. Conversely, one's individual development is not only reflected in a "psychic" character or personality structure. The body is also the carrier and expression of the individual biography; it has and *knows* its own history. This is what we may call *body memory*: from birth onwards, the experiences that the child has with people and things are sedimented as behavioral patterns, skills, and habits (Fuchs 2012a). This bodily memory, implicitly effective in every action and behavior, constitutes the individual habitus of a person, his personal way of living in the world and of dealing with others.

The person is formed in and through his body; he appears in it more and more clearly and individually. His being is continual becoming, and this becoming is increasingly a doing. The body is therefore not a shell behind which the person is hidden and is indicated only symbolically. Rather, a person's attitudes, behavior, and habits are always simultaneously attitudes, movement patterns and dispositions of their body—right down to the characteristic style of gait, gestures, and facial expressions, articulation, and prosody. We recognize a person by his posture and behavior; his corporeality is part of his personality, his identity. Not only "inner," psychological or mental characteristics but also the individual body constitutes the person.

We are therefore embodied persons for each other, too. We do not perceive the other as a material object from whose outer movements we infer an "inhabitant" within, hidden as in a capsule. The body is rather the living, animated appearance of the person; in it the person presents and manifests himself. In his gaze I see *the other person himself*; taking his hand in greeting, I give *the other* my hand, and in his words I hear *the person himself*. If the person were somewhere inside the body, we would only see empty glances and instead of words we would only hear sounds in which no one speaks and which we must suppose to be signs of an inaccessible inner world. Persons, however, are the *primordial phenomenon*: that which shows itself and which is itself present in its appearance.

Interpersonality

The identification of personhood and brain becomes completely absurd once we consider the person in their constitutive relationality, i.e., in social relationships. A person's family and kinship relationships, her social roles, such as gender, profession, or status, are inseparably linked to the concept of the person. It is no coincidence that the word "person" itself originates from the world of theatre—as is well known, the ancient *persona* was the theatrical mask or role and, derived from this, the role of an individual in society. Whether this relationality is understood in a radical way, as in Buber or Löwith—i.e., the person only becomes a person as such through participation in social relationships—or whether it is simply regarded as a key feature of personhood, the concept is certainly not restricted to the individual: "To be a person is to occupy a place within a field where other people have their places" (Spaemann 2006: 182). Persons only exist in the plural. And personal identity rests not on a self-sufficient inwardness but is necessarily of a relational nature: "I do not have to search very far for others: I find them in my experience" (Merleau-Ponty 1973: 138–9), namely in the relationship patterns, modes of reaction, and preferences that make up my personality; "we are in no way locked inside ourselves" (Merleau-Ponty 1973: 139).

The intersubjective nature of the person applies in equal measure to the characteristic that is often regarded as special proof of one's individuality, namely self-consciousness. This too is an achievement that requires community and interaction with others. "I exist only in communication with the other," writes Jaspers; "a single isolated consciousness would be without communication, without question and answer, therefore without *self*-consciousness […] it must recognize itself in the other self" (Jaspers 1973: 50, 55; trans. T. F.). This already applies to development in early childhood: in the course of the first year of life, the infant first learns to grasp that others are "like me" by imitating them and communicating with them prelingually (Trevarthen 2001; Meltzoff/Prinz 2002). Recognizing oneself in others in this way is a prerequisite for the ability to take others' perspectives and to self-reflect which children acquire in the course of further practical and linguistic interactions: they learn to see themselves through the eyes of others (Tomasello 1999, 2008; Fuchs 2013).

This interactive dynamic is permanently reflected in the structure of personhood, inasmuch as a developed self-consciousness has internalized the relationships with others but still contains intersubjectivity *as a constitutive moment*. Because the self-relationship implies the capacity to see oneself from the perspective of the "generalized other" (Mead 1934) and to speak to oneself as someone else would speak to you. In this sense, Plato already understood thoughts as "the inner conversation of the soul with itself, which goes on without a voice" (*Sophist* 263e; Plato 1997). The mobility of perspective and the ability to reflect are thus the result of an originally interactive movement—as it were, an organized reflection of experiences of interaction. In this respect, the basic structure of personhood is not to be understood in a purely individualistic or substantialistic way but only as a dynamic, open structure: self-consciousness is a "self-talk" that always implicitly includes others. It is obvious that this complex, self-referential, and intersubjective structure of self-awareness eludes a reduction to local brain activities, even if brain research likes to talk about "self-models," or "self-modules," and corresponding brain areas.[5]

Critique of Localizationism

The previous criticism of the cerebral subject was directed at the category mistake of identifying one part with the whole, namely the brain with the person. Bennett and Hacker (2003) have called it the *mereological fallacy*. The psychiatrist Erwin Straus once put it succinctly: "It is man who thinks, not the brain" (Straus 1956: 112). But what do we then see in the colorful brain-imaging pictures on which certain structures show increased neuronal activity? Do they not at least show us the material correlates of our mental processes?

Here we are dealing with a second, *localization fallacy*, namely the identification of conscious activities with local brain processes: in the visual cortex, supposedly visual perceptions are produced, in the amygdala fear, in the temporal lobe memories. There are always new areas for all kinds of psychic phenomena—pain, grief, empathy, malicious joy, racial prejudice, conscious deception, even personality traits. This research program is primarily based on neuroimaging which, so to speak, represents the specific brain activities in vivo. The suggestive images of brain activity "when perceiving," "when feeling," or "thinking" make it all too easy to identify such activities with local neuronal processes.

---

[5] See for example Blakeslee (1996) on the "self-module"; Metzinger (1999) on the "self-model." Lindemann (2007: 407 ff.) discusses the inherent limits of the modeling of self-consciousness by brain research.

Critique of Neuroimaging

But the evidence of the pictures is deceptive. First of all, the techniques do not measure neuronal activity itself but only indirect parameters. In functional magnetic resonance imaging (fMRI), for example, it is the increased blood flow and oxygen consumption in certain areas of the brain. In fact, these are not "images of the brain" at all, but rather visualizations of statistical constructs formed from the average values gleaned from (usually) about 10 to 20 test persons, since it is almost impossible to obtain meaningful results individually due to the extremely small differences in activity. In addition, the basic activity of the brain is determined in advance and then subtracted from the measured values to ensure that only the locally increased activity levels appear in the image. Of course, it is by no means clear whether the experiential phenomena investigated actually correspond to the most active brain structures. The brain is undeniably regionally specialized, i.e., different areas and centers fulfill different functions. However, at the same time, every other region of the brain (where nothing seems to happen during functional imaging) is active and participating in different ways in the overall experience.

What the images actually show and what happens in the brain when we experience something actually requires careful interpretation. In addition, the recordings made in brain research are created in laboratory situations, and the relationships between the processes of consciousness and the environmental context, along with their temporal sequence, are usually ignored. These aspects—relationality, intentionality, and temporality—are however essential characteristics of consciousness. If one takes all these methodical limitations together, then data on the brain's local metabolic activities can to a certain extent reveal its functional specialization, but can provide no more than *indicators* for psychological processes. Figuratively speaking: you only see the smoke, not the fire, and even of the smoke only a snapshot.

So, if brain researchers nevertheless claim that they are able to "read thoughts" in the brain (Haynes et al. 2007; Haynes 2012), it must first be stated that metabolic processes are not thoughts. Granted, it is now technologically possible to assign the specific distribution of brain activity to certain categories of objects, colors, or similar things that a person is thinking about at any specific moment. For this purpose, the objects are first presented to the person repeatedly, then the data collected in the fMRI are averaged by intensive computer processing in such a way that it is highly probable that one of several alternative thought contents can be deduced from the activity patterns. The same applies to the possible differentiation of simple thought operations such as adding versus subtracting, affirming or negating (cf. Schleim 2008: 84 ff.). However, these are always only correlations that have already been established according to the statements of the test persons, and that do not go beyond rather rough categorizations—again, it is not possible to actually follow thoughts.

Holism of Consciousness

But, apart from the methodological problems mentioned previously, there is an even more fundamental fallacy hidden in the localization of conscious activities, because none of the respective specialized regions is in a position to achieve the complex integration that is the basis of consciousness. On the contrary, each subjective experience always involves a network of neuronal assemblies that extends over the entire brain, and this in the closest connection with the rest of the organism. This also corresponds to the complexity of the experience itself: every specific description of functions, such as seeing, hearing, thinking, feeling, etc., isolate single functions of consciousness while actual subjective experiences always remain holistic. Each of our perceptions is not only embedded in a bodily background experience but also connected with feelings, memories, and language concepts. There is no "pure" pain, no "pure" seeing or hearing. Conscious experience is not composed of partial components; it is primarily a uniform process that is differentiated into specific activities and functions according to the requirements of the situation.

Therefore, the talk of "neuronal correlates of the mental state X" is misleading: it implies that phenomena such as perceptions, feelings, or thought processes can be isolated from the conscious experience as a whole. However, these phenomena are not separable states but require a *subject* who perceives, feels, and thinks. But what the "correlate" of this subject is, which brain centers and activities are necessary for it, and whether it does not involve the entire organism beyond the brain, cannot be decided at all with the help of imaging studies. By determining local differences in activity, therefore, a mental state as such has neither been localized nor identified with neuronal processes.[6]

We see that even the ever-growing research into the functional specialization of the brain does not allow us to conclude that there is a localization of conscious activities as such. Consciousness is not a local but an *integral* function of the organism, as long as the latter is linked to its environment in constant interactions. This concept is presented in the following overview.[7]

---

[6] For a critique of the concept of "neural correlates of consciousness" see also Noë and Thompson (2004).

[7] Cf. my detailed description in *Ecology of the Brain* (Fuchs 2018).

Personhood as Embodied Subjectivity

We will not find our experiences in the brain, nor even sufficient neuronal correlates for them, as indispensable as brain activity is. So, how is the relationship between person and brain to be adequately understood?

We said that the human being thinks, feels, perceives, and acts, not the brain. And the human being is first of all a living organism, a being of flesh and blood. This also corresponds to the classical understanding of the person as a body-mind unit. Persons exist only as embodied subjects, that is, as *living beings*.

However, for the current neurosciences, the body plays a very subordinate role. It remains a kind of physiological carrying device for the brain, in which the incorporeal inner world of consciousness is supposed to arise. But this "cerebrocentrism" neglects the interrelationships and circuits in which the brain is situated—as if one were to examine the heart without the circulation or examine the lungs without the respiratory cycle. The reason for this is that the neurosciences have no concept of a living organism. They are still trapped in the computer metaphor of the mind, as if consciousness could jump out of neuronal computational processes were they sufficiently complex. What is missing here was already recognized in the nineteenth century by Ludwig Feuerbach:

> It is neither the soul which thinks and senses [...], nor the brain; for the brain is a *physiological abstraction*—an organ removed from the totality, separated from the skull, face, and body as a whole, and fixed for itself. But the brain is only an organ of thought as long as it is connected with a human head and body. (Feuerbach 1846/1967: 177; trans. T. F.)

So, only the living person can think and feel. In the last two decades, a new direction has developed in the cognitive- and neurosciences that brings these interrelationships to the fore, the paradigm of *embodied cognition*.[8] It regards subjectivity as embodied in the entire organism and as embedded in the environment. Consciousness is therefore not located in the brain, but extends over the perceived body into the environment that is relevant for us in each case.

Brain, Body, and Environment

How can we imagine this in more detail? Conscious experience is based on two continuous interactions, namely a) between brain and body and b) between brain, body, and environment.

a) All consciousness is based primarily on the constant interaction of the brain with the rest of the organism, that means, on the signals from the limbs,

---

[8] See in particular Varela et al. (1991); Gallagher (2005); Thompson (2007); Di Paolo et al. (2017) and many others.

muscles, heart, circulation, and intestines, not least on the biochemical milieu of blood and cerebrospinal fluid in which the brain is embedded. Signals from these peripheral systems are processed in the brainstem, diencephalon, and higher brain centers, while conversely, neuronal and neuro-endocrine signals constantly regulate the periphery and the internal milieu of the body. This circular interaction of the brain and the entire organism forms the basis for a *bodily background experience* that always accompanies us whatever we are currently perceiving, thinking, or doing (Fuchs 2012b). It is "the feeling of life itself" (Damasio 1994: 150), with the hue of well-being or discomfort, pleasure or displeasure, freshness or exhaustion, and other basic moods that already contain a pre-*reflexive self-experience*, a "what-it-is-likeness."

The primordial feelings of being alive "reflect the current state of the body along varied dimensions, for example, along the scale that ranges from pleasure to pain, and they originate at the level of the brain stem rather than the cerebral cortex" (Damasio 2010: 21). It is true that our attention is mostly focused on perceptions, imaginations, or thoughts, which can lead us to believe that these functions are the actual activity of consciousness. But all higher intentional performances always remain embedded in the basal bodily self-experience. The maintenance of homeostasis, i.e., of the inner milieu and thus of the viability of the organism, is the primary function of consciousness, as manifested in instinct, hunger, thirst, lust, or aversion. We can also formulate it in this way: *processes of life and processes of experience* ("Leben" and "Erleben") *are inseparably linked.*[9] As conscious beings, we are at the same time living, embodied beings.

In the same way, the *emotions* that are at the core of our subjective experience are linked to the interaction between the brain and the rest of the organism, which is primarily mediated via the hypothalamus. Moods and feelings are, from a biological point of view, always states of the whole organism, which include almost all subsystems of the body: central and peripheral nervous system, hormonal system, heart, circulation, respiration, viscera, facial, and gestural expression muscles. It is not possible to experience anxiety without feeling a bodily tension or trembling, without the beating of the heart or shortness of breath, and the same applies to anger, joy, or sadness. Every feeling is inseparably linked to changes in the body landscape, and without this *bodily resonance* we could not experience feelings in the full sense (Damasio 1999; Fuchs 2018: 120 ff.). Thus, even our basal consciousness and feelings by no means rest solely on neuronal processes in the neocortex but extend rather to the whole body.

---

[9] On this, see Thompson (2007: 128 ff.).

b) Let us now move on to sensorimotor interactions with the environment, the basis of our being in the world. Every perception and action also requires the body, but not only as an apparatus for signal transmission or movement execution, also because only the sensitive and mobile body also conveys the *unity* of perception and movement. Jakob von Uexküll (1920/1973) spoke of the sensorimotor "functional circle": what a living being perceives is always dependent on its movement and vice versa. This applies to the movements of the hand that touches an object as well as to the scanning of objects with the moving gaze: in seeing, the actual or possible movement of one's own body is always taken into account (Noë 2004). We perceive actively, i.e., we look at, listen to, feel for. Perception is therefore not merely an internal state of the brain but a continuous bodily interaction with the environment.

Actions are of course even more embodied: when I speak, this is not only based on a motor program in my brain, but also on the constant feedback of my throat muscles, on hearing my own voice, and the reactions of listeners. Speaking, just like grasping or dancing, is not an ability or activity of the brain, but that of an embodied subject. In general, the brain and its networks provide "open loops," as it were, which are then closed by the body and suitable objects in the environment to form the respective sensorimotor circle.

Conscious experience therefore only arises *in the overarching system of organism and environment*, through the interplay of many components to which the brain and the entire body with its organs, senses, and limbs belong, just as much as the appropriate objects of the environment. The brain is the organ that mediates these interactions, in short: an organ of *mediation and relation*. But, in the brain itself there is no experiencing, no consciousness, no thoughts. For comparison, one can think of another central life function, namely breathing: can we find it inside the lungs? Certainly not—respiration is not localizable in any single place. It is the entire process in which the organism takes in ambient air, transforms it, and gives it out again, an exchange and circular process, in other words, which would not be possible without the environment, the respiratory organs, the blood circulation, and the metabolism of oxygen and carbon dioxide in the entire organism. The lung too is a relational organ that can only perform its function embedded in circular processes.

The same applies to consciousness. It is not to be found in one single place; it is not an inner image of the world in the brain but is itself the living process of our embodied interaction with the world. The brain is indispensable for conscious experience, because all the previously mentioned circular processes are linked together in it—comparable to the tracks that converge in a main railway station. Without the main station, train traffic would certainly collapse, as would conscious experience without a brain. Nevertheless, to continue the comparison, *train traffic is neither generated by the station nor can it be located there*. Instead, traffic uses the track system with its many connections, crossings, and its central coordination point in the main station so that everything runs as smoothly as possible, and people reach their destinations. In the same way, the activity of consciousness represents the "ecological integral" of the entire relationship between brain, organization, and environment: consciousness is being in the world.

Brain Transplantation

Finally, the organismic embodiment of the subject also sheds critical light on the thought experiment of brain transplantation. The person's implied identification with the brain is based on the assumption that his identity consists of nothing more than his psychological dispositions, memories, and knowledge as stored in the neuronal structures of the brain. The transplantation argument thus pre-supposes a Cartesian, disembodied view of the person. But as we saw, selfhood consists primarily in a pre-reflexive, bodily background feeling, which is not based on neuronal processes in the cerebral cortex but on the life process of the entire organism. The embedding of the brain in biochemical, neuroendocrine, and humoral processes of vital self-regulation cannot be understood according to the pattern of digital information processing in a computer. However, it is from these circular, living processes that basal self-experience results.

What is presupposed in the transplantation thought experiment, namely the continuity of phenomenal self-awareness after brain transplantation, is therefore anything but self-evident. We do not know in the slightest what the consequences of a separation of brain and body and thus an interruption of the continuity of life and experience would be. It is highly questionable whether the conscious functions would regenerate at all after the brain stem has been separated from the spinal cord and reimplanted in a new body. For a successful transplantation, the complex feedback loops between brain and body would also have to be precisely restored at the vital and sensorimotor level. And, even then, serious disturbances of self-experience would have to be expected, because the entire endocrine, autonomic, interoceptive, and emotional reactions of the foreign body would no longer match the neuronal dispositions of the brain. A severe self-alienation and disorientation up to psychotic confusion would be the most likely consequence.

Moreover, every bodily ability based on procedural bodily memory—walking, grasping, or speaking, not to mention playing the piano or other complex abilities—are tied to highly subtle brain-body co-ordinations and would all have to be relearned. Finally, let us think of the disturbing effects on one's experience of identity that would be expected from suddenly having a foreign body shape, a different voice, a foreign face, and the alienated reactions of our friends and acquaintances. All of these factors only allow the conclusion to be drawn that a brain transplant would not preserve the identity of the person, but would at best create a new, severely disturbed individual who would not have any clear continuity with either the donor or the recipient of the transplant. The person is embodied in the organism as a whole, and a separation of brain and body would not preserve but destroy the person.[10]

Conclusion

If neurobiology wants to look inside the person, it is looking in the wrong place. Not that neuronal processes are dispensable for conscious experience—on the contrary. But they are not the place where we find the consciousness and self-hood of a person. A person feels, sees, thinks, and acts—not the brain, not the mind or the consciousness. We are neither brains nor minds but living beings, embodied and visible in our bodies. There is no second version of ourselves ex-isting in our brains or in our minds.[11]

The brain has neither mental states nor consciousness, because the brain *does not live*—it is only the *organ* of a living being, or a living person. Thought ex-periments about a brain in a vat or a brain transplant can be set aside: only a brain that is connected to a sentient and mobile body is able to serve as a central organ for mental processes, because only through the constant interactions of brain, body, and environment can the structures of conscious experience be created and stabilized.

It is therefore wrong to identify the subject or person with the brain and to search for the "personal" there. What constitutes persons essentially is their embodiment, their aliveness, as well as their being in relationships, and these living, intentional, and social relationships to the world are neither products of the brain nor to be found in it. Undoubtedly the abilities of the person as well as the realization of these abilities as conscious expressions of a life are closely tied

---

[10] For a critique of the thought experiment of the "brain in a vat" see Chapter 4 in this volume.

[11] Cf. also Merleau-Ponty (1962: xii): "... there is no inner man, man is in the world, and only in the world does he know himself." Merleau-Ponty here refers critically to Augustine's con-cept of "*intus hominis*," admittedly not to negate the possibility of inner self-reflection, but rather to reject the idea that one encounters a Cartesian mind or one's "actual self" in re-flection. After all, the personal pronoun "I" does not refer to an "I"—this is a philosopher's invention—but to the respective speaker, i.e., to an embodied *person*. The same applies to self-reflection: it is the reflection of a living being, not of a mind on itself. In this respect, brain research, when it searches for the person or subject in the brain, ultimately remains bound to the inner-world paradigm of Cartesianism.

to brain functions. The brain is therefore a crucial condition of the possibility of personal existence in the world. However, the person is not a part of the body, but the body-mind unity, the living human being. Persons have brains, they are not their brains.

References

Bennett, M. R., P. M. S. Hacker. 2003. *Philosophical Foundations of Neuroscience*: Oxford: Blackwell Publishing.

Blakeslee, T. 1996. *Beyond the Conscious Mind: Unlocking the Secrets of the Self*. New York: Plenum Press.

Choudhury, S., J. Slaby (eds.) 2012. *Critical Neuroscience: A Handbook of the Social and Cultural Contexts of Neuroscience*. London: Wiley-Blackwell.

Damasio, A. 1994. *Descartes's Error: Emotion, Reason and the Human Brain*. London: Picador.

Damasio, A. 1999. *The Feeling of What Happens: Body and Emotion in the Making of Consciousness*. New York: Hartcourt Brace & Co.

Damasio, A. 2010. *Self Comes to Mind: Constructing the Conscious Brain*. New York: Pantheon Books.

Di Paolo, E., T. Buhrmann, X. Barandiaran. 2017. *Sensorimotor Life: An Enactive Proposal*. Oxford: Oxford University Press.

Eagleman, D. 2015. *Incognito: The Secret Lives of the Brain*. New York: Pantheon Books.

Feuerbach, L. 1967. "Wider den Dualismus von Leib und Seele, Fleisch und Geist." In A. Schmidt (ed.) *Anthropologischer Materialismus. Ausgewählte Schriften I*. Frankfurt/M., Berlin: Europäische Verlags-Anstalt (pp. 165–191). (First published 1846.)

Fuchs, T. 2011. "The brain—a mediating organ." *Journal of Consciousness Studies* **18**: 196–221.

Fuchs, T. 2012a. "The feeling of being alive. Organic foundations of self-awareness." In J. Fingerhut, S. Marienberg (eds.) *Feelings of Being Alive*. Berlin: De Gruyter (pp. 149–166).

Fuchs, T. 2012b. "The phenomenology of body memory." In S. Koch., T. Fuchs, M. Summa, C. Müller. (eds.) *Body Memory, Metaphor and Movement*. John Benjamins, Amsterdam (pp. 9–22).

Fuchs, T. 2013. "The phenomenology and development of social perspectives." *Phenomenology and the Cognitive Sciences* **12**: 655–683.

Fuchs, T. 2018. *Ecology of the Brain: The Phenomenology and Biology of the Embodied Mind*. Oxford, Oxford University Press.

Gallagher, S. 2005. *How the Body Shapes the Mind*. New York: Clarendon Press.

Gazzaniga, M. S. 2005. *The Ethical Brain*. New York: Dana Press.

Haynes, J. D., K. Sakai, G. Rees, S. Gilbert, C. Frith, R. E. Passingham. 2007. "Reading hidden intentions in the human brain." *Current Biology* **17**: 323–328.

Haynes, J. D. 2012. "Brain reading." In S. Richmond, G. Rees, S. J. Edwards (eds.) *I Know What You're Thinking: Brain Imaging and Mental Privacy*. Oxford: Oxford University Press (pp. 29–40).

Jaspers, K. 1973. *Philosophie II: Existenzerhellung.* Berlin, Heidelberg, New York: Springer.

Leibniz, G. W. 2009. *The Monadology and Other Philosophical Writing.* R. Latta (trans.) Ithaca/NY: Cornell University Library. (Monadology first published 1714.) http://home.datacomm.ch/kerguelen/monadology/printable.html

Lindemann, G. 2007. "Plädoyer für einen methodologisch pluralistischen Monismus." In H.-P. Krüger (ed.) *Hirn als Subjekt? Philosophische Grenzfragen der Neurobiologie.* Berlin: Akademie-Verlag (pp. 401–410).

Locke, J. 1689/1997. *An Essay Concerning Human Understanding.* London: Penguin. (Originally Published 1689.)

Mead, G. H. 1934. *Mind, Self, and Society from the Standpoint of a Social Behaviorist.* Chicago: University of Chicago Press.

Meltzoff, A. N., W. Prinz. (Hg.) 2002. *The Imitative Mind: Development, Evolution, and Brain Bases.* Cambridge: Cambridge University Press.

Merleau-Ponty, M. 1962. *Phenomenology of Perception.* C. Smith (trans.) London New York: Routledge.

Merleau-Ponty, M. 1973. *Adventures of the Dialectic.* J. Bien (trans.) Evanstone: Northwestern University Press.

Metzinger, T. 1999. *Subjekt und Selbstmodell.* 2nd edn. Paderborn: Mentis.

Metzinger, T. 2009. *The Ego Tunnel: The Science of the Mind and the Myth of the Self.* New York: Basic Books.

Nagel, T. 1974. "What is it like to be a bat?" *The Philosophical Review* **83**: 435–450.

Noë, A. 2004. *Action in Perception.* Cambridge, MA: MIT Press.

Noë, A., E. Thompson. 2004. "Are there neural correlates of consciousness?" *Journal of Consciousness Studies* **11**: 3–28.

Plato. 1997. "Sophist" In **John M Cooper** (ed.) *Collected Works.* Cambridge: Hackett (pp. 235–293).

Putnam, H. 1981. *Reason, Truth, and History.* Cambridge: Cambridge University Press.

Schleim, S. 2008. *Gedankenlesen: Pionierarbeit der Hirnforschung.* Hannover: Heise.

Schmitz, H. 1995. *Der unerschöpfliche Gegenstand. Grundzüge der Philosophie.* 2. Aufl. Bonn: Bouvier.

Slaby, J. 2010. "Steps towards a critical neuroscience." *Phenomenology and the Cognitive Sciences* **9**: 397–416.

Spaemann, R. 2006. *Persons: The Difference Between "Someone" and "Something".* O. O'Donovan (trans.) Oxford: Oxford University Press.

Straus, E. 1956. *Vom Sinn der Sinne.* 2nd edn. Berlin: Springer.

Thompson, E. 2007. *Mind in Life: Biology, Phenomenology, and the Sciences of Mind.* Cambridge, MA: Harvard University Press.

Tomasello, M. 1999. *The Cultural Origins of Human Cognition.* Cambridge, MA: Harvard University Press.

Tomasello, M. 2008. *Origins of Human Communication.* Cambridge, MA: MIT Press.

Trevarthen, C. 2001. "The neurobiology of early communication: Intersubjective regulations in human brain development." In A. F. Kalverboer, A. Gramsberg (eds.) *Handbook of Brain and Behavior in Human Development.* Dordrecht, Boston, London: Kluwer (pp. 841–881).

Uexküll, J. V. 1973. *Theoretische Biologie.* Frankfurt/M.: Suhrkamp. (First published 1920.)

Varela, F. J., E. Thompson, E. Rosch. 1991. *The Embodied Mind: Cognitive Science and Human Experience*. Cambridge, MA: MIT Press.

Vidal, F. 2011. "Von unserem eigenen Gehirn überlebt." In C. M. Schmitz, L. Kesner (eds.) *Images of the Mind. Bildwelten des Geistes aus Kunst und Wissenschaft*. Dresden: Wallstein Verlag (pp. 41–48).

Chapter 5

Embodied Freedom: A Libertarian Position

Introduction

The freedom to decide and act is a primary experience of our everyday life. Kant wrote in 1783:

> In fact, the practical concept of freedom has nothing to do with the speculative concept, which is abandoned entirely to metaphysicians. For I can be quite indifferent as to the origin of my state in which I am now to act; I ask only what I now have to do, and then freedom is a necessary practical presupposition [...]. Even the most obstinate skeptic grants that, when it comes to acting, all sophistical scruples about a universally deceptive illusion must come to nothing. In the same way, the most confirmed fatalist, who is a fatalist as long as he gives himself up to mere speculation, must still, as soon as he has to do with wisdom and duty, always act as if he were free, and this idea also actually produces the deed that accords with it and can alone produce it. It is hard to cease altogether to be human. (Kant 1783/1999: 10)

Kant thus formulates the irrefutable experience of practical freedom. Even if we were to come to the conclusion on the basis of philosophical considerations or scientific findings that freedom of will is an illusion, this illusion would not be dispelled. On the contrary, the agony of choice often enough shows us that we cannot escape the decision, that we are, as Sartre put it, even "condemned to freedom." The option of determinism thus ultimately remains an academic one—we cannot *act* according to it.

But we can go even further. It is almost a basic condition of our everyday dealings with each other that we do not regard ourselves and others as completely determined by physical causes. Moral feelings such as guilt, remorse, indignation, blame, or gratitude would be lost if it could be proven that the actions to which they are directed really originated from blind physical events. We consider and treat each other as persons, i.e., as beings who are not simply at the mercy of internal impulses or biological processes, but who are able to suspend their primary drives, to pause and weigh up, to determine, and to direct their actions according to reasons. Not only criminal law but even our everyday expectations and mutual claims are based on this prerequisite. From this follows: "A complete naturalistic description and explanation of human behavior

In Defense of the Human Being. Thomas Fuchs, Oxford University Press. © Suhrkamp Verlag 2021.
DOI: 10.1093/oso/9780192898197.003.0006

is incompatible with our morality in the life-world" (Nida-Rümelin 2005: 33; trans. T. F.).

These introductory these are not intended to justify the reality of freedom, but *to assign the burden of proof*, which in a centuries-old philosophical dispute such as the freedom of the will, can already be decisive. Anyone who claims that the possibility of human freedom has been refuted by scientific research or philosophical arguments, I argue, bears the burden of proof. Because he is liable to challenge us with a serious inconsistency between practical experience and theoretical convictions, which we are supposed to somehow reconcile; this of course would only be possible by means of a blatant "as-if," or a virtualization of our primary experience.

I do not consider the denial of freedom in the strong sense to be convincing and would like, in what follows, to advocate a libertarian conception, i.e., to defend the intuition of freedom within practical experience against its determinist opponents. I do not claim to solve all the problems of freedom of will, for example, to give a final answer to how we should picture the connection between our voluntary decisions and actions and neurophysiological processes. It must suffice to show there are no convincing empirical or philosophical arguments against the legitimacy of our experience of freedom.

However, I want to avoid from the outset an unfruitful alternative in the debate, which still follows a predetermined dualistic path. On the one side, there is the body apparatus subject to purely physical laws, including the brain, on the other there is the intelligible, rational world of the mind. Depending on the point of view, one side should then determine the other; either "the brain" or "the I" should make the decisions. What remains outside the scope of this approach is that decisions belong first and foremost to the conduct of life. Deciding is not an isolated and instantaneous act of will, but a more or less extended, "maturing" process. This process, however, does not only involve conscious considerations and reasons but also pre- and unconscious motives, feelings, intuitions, expectations, experiences, and ultimately the entire personal life story of the acting person.

In place of the dualism of rational subject or brain as decisive authority I would therefore like to put the concept of *embodied or personal freedom*. The person is not something composed of mind and body but is above all a living being, i.e., a psychophysical unity, and in this respect its decisions are also life processes in which the mental, emotional and intellectual components interact with each other. If one wants to find the cause of a person's actions one must not look for them in an "I" or in the brain but only in the person as a whole with all their mental and physical states, or in other words, in the person as an embodied subjectivity.

I would like to elaborate on this thesis in the following. I will start with a conceptual clarification of the question whether decisions can be meaningfully attributed to a physiological subsystem such as the brain. From this a number of preconditions arise, on the basis of which an embodied libertarian concept of freedom will be developed. In the third section I turn to some scientific and philosophical objections to such a concept of freedom.

Can Brains make Decisions?

According to the naturalistic position, brain processes work deterministically, and we cannot do anything other than what our brain determines. In fact, decisions are ultimately directed by unconscious sub-personal processes, and our actions are then triggered by the premotor areas of brain, before we become conscious of them. Thus, the brain only deludes us into believing we are acting and responsible persons, when in fact we can only ratify the brain's decisions retrospectively.

> [. . .] our actions are clearly the result of a causal chain of neuronal activity in premotor and motor areas of the brain. [. . .] although we may experience that our conscious decisions and thoughts cause our actions, these experiences are in fact based on readouts of brain activity in a network of brain areas that control voluntary action. (Haggard 2011)

> [. . .] our brains have to function as efficient, unconscious computers that nevertheless make rational decisions. (Swaab 2014: 331).

So, do brains make decisions? Let's take a chess computer for comparison and set up the pieces in a certain way to find out whether move A or move B is the more favorable in this position. By means of a programmed algorithm the computer calculates the result: move B.[1] Should we now say that the computer has made a decision for B? Of course not, because the possibility of calculating move A never existed in reality. The result B was fixed from the beginning at the moment of input, not unlike the solution of a complex equation, and only the fact that the electrical process took place in finite time due to its complexity could suggest something like a progressive "decision process"—as if the apparatus had hesitated and then decided. So, the alternative "A or B" was *only in our minds*—as soon as we set the program in motion, it was over.

---

[1] For the sake of simplicity, think of an endgame in which the computer can actually calculate all moves completely until it reaches the optimal move. But even an artificial neural network, which calculates and "evaluates" the more complex sequences of the game in middle phases by means of synaptic weightings, does not change the blindness of these calculations.

Here we encounter a constituent of the concept of decision, namely that of *counterfactual possibility*. To decide requires being able to bracket the merely factual and to think of the possible alternatives *as possibilities*—I could do this or not, or something else. This is the prerequisite for the fact that there is an alternative to every ability to act, or at least the possibility of omission. "For when acting depends on us, not acting does so too, and when saying no does so, saying yes does too," Aristotle already saw (*Nicomachean Ethics*: 1113b7; Aristotle 2002: 130). The prerequisite for freedom of decision is therefore first of all a space of thinking, of possibilities, in which we are able to move free from factual constraints. We can imagine the possible by suspending the immediate reality, so to speak. The human mind is essentially characterized by *negation*, that is, by the ability to think not only A but also non-A, an either/or, and the irrealis: could, had, would. But negation, not-being and thus possibility *as such* does not exist in physical nature, as Sartre famously argued in *Being and Nothingness*. Negation is equally absent from the digital world of the computer. For computers, there is indeed no possibility, and therefore they do not decide anything, no matter how much time they need for calculation. Even a random number generator would not change this—we would not say, for instance, that a lottery machine has made the decision for the number 12 today.

Now one might object that brains work completely differently than computers. That is correct, but that is not the point here: if the neuroscientist views neuronal processes as purely physically determined processes, then the number of variables is larger, but the result is no less predestined (even if we could not predict it). Thus, for example, when I decided whether I would rather go to the cinema or work on my chapter, there was never any other possibility than the one I actually realized. The concept of decision, however, presupposes the existence of alternative possibilities for a subject, namely the presentation of a future to which I can give or withhold my consent. In contrast, since my brain could not do more than make me write, and the possibility of going to the cinema never existed *at the level of neural description*, the brain has not made a decision.

Conclusion: an exclusively scientific description of the world, in which no subjects of ideas, desires, and evaluations occur, makes the concept of possibility and thus the concept of decision meaningless. The possible, that is, the non-existence that we can imagine and choose in our decision, cannot be found in the merely factual. If the perspective of the subject is ruled out as illusionary or irrelevant, then there has never been any other possibility than the factual event: brains do not decide.

Of course, neither is it a fictitious "ego" or an immaterial spirit that makes the decision. To decide and to act means a self-determination which can only be meaningfully attributed to the organism as a whole, or to the embodied person.

The brain should then be understood as the organ by means of which the organism wins a space of freedom and controls itself. "But it would be inappropriate to speak of the brain making the decision, because this would identify the *organ* of self-control with the *execution of the control performance*, whose subject is the organism as a whole, i.e., the organically embodied subject" (Lindemann 2007: 261). Rationalist philosophers set their sights too high, so to speak, and assign the decision to the subjective mind. Neuro-determinists, on the other hand, set them too low; they go below the level at which decision-making actually takes place, which is not in the brain but *as the life conduct of the embodied person*. The brain is an organ of freedom, but it is only its organ, not its subject—brains do not decide.

Freedom as a Personal Ability

The proof of this actually trivial truth has at least brought us an important result: free decisions presuppose the ability to imagine and anticipate the possible as such; they thus proceed in a *space of possibility*, of an open future. This space is opened up by an *inhibition*: we have the ability to suspend our own impulses and desires, to pause and to examine whether and to what extent we want to transform them into actions.[2] Often this pausing also results from ambiguous or multi-valent situations in which different competing possibilities present themselves. These are also situations of more or less pronounced disorientation, a crisis (Greek *krísis* = "conflict," "decision"). The inhibition or interruption of the unreflected movement of life now opens up a *moratorium*, a more or less extended period of time for the process of reflection, deliberation, of articulating and clarifying motives and reasons. In virtual test movements, the individual anticipates future possibilities, their advantages, risks, or obstacles, in order to find a new coherence and orientation.

Of course, this is not a strictly systematic but rather a dynamic and creative process in which conscious and unconscious components, feelings, desires, ideas, expectations, and reasons influence and drive each other forward. Therefore, the result cannot be derived from pre-existing determinants. We are neither dealing with a vector addition of independent, pre-fixed motivations nor with a rational calculation or algorithm of reasons. Rather, the various

---

2 John Locke already noted (1690/1997: 242 (Book 2: § 47)): "For the mind having in most cases, as is evident in experience, a power to *suspend* the execution and satisfaction of any of its desires, and so all, one after another, is at liberty to consider the objects of them; examine them on all sides and weigh them with others. In this lies the liberty man has [...]. We have a power to *suspend* the prosecution of this or that desire, as everyone daily may experiment in himself."

components enter into the open space of possibility and are set in a free play that takes the form of an inner dialogue, a *self-relationship*. This is now the central prerequisite of freedom: by placing ourselves in a relationship with them, our motives, wishes, and reasons do not simply remain what they are but instead enter, as it were, an inner stage on which we can weigh and evaluate them. In this way, we gain the freedom to take a stance toward them and ultimately to make a choice. The self-relationship thus fundamentally transforms what happens. If the process of deliberating and deciding were only a linear sequence of the components involved, we would have no influence on the result. The freedom of choice is based on a consulting of oneself, on the self-relation of the person.[3]

The neurobiological experiments used to address the question of free will, in particular the Libet experiment and its successors (Libet 1985), focus on movement triggers or choice reactions that occur in fractions of a second. This focusing misses the phenomenon, as it were, by looking too closely. Freedom in a relevant sense is bound to a time-spanning process of will formation, which cannot be broken down into arbitrarily short partial moments. The paradigm of free decisions is therefore not the arbitrary choice reaction tasks of neurobiological experiments, but rather practical life decisions. "What suits me?," "What is really important to me?," "Who do I want to be?"—these are questions that arise in such situations. They serve to *explicate* a way of life that otherwise represents the implicit background of life, but is not yet differentiated into specific directions or goals. The future relevance of this phase is not sufficiently described by the consideration of future possibilities. Anticipation also implies a kind of "feeling-in-advance" or a bodily felt sense: "How I will feel when I do this."

Successful decisions therefore require an affective bodily sense of intuition, in which previous experience is implicitly involved.[4] Deciding now means approaching a feeling of "fittingness" or congruence between the imagined possibilities and an updated conception of oneself, which contains one's own motives, experiences, preferences, and wishes. In the ongoing process of clarification, actively seeking, cognitive and passively receptive, intuitive moments

---

[3] Of course, this dialogical self-relationship cannot be understood without an at least implicit intersubjectivity: in our deliberations and decisions there is always something like an inner witness to whom we could report and account for our motives and actions, an *implicit other*. The responsibility for our decisions is therefore not only created by a subsequent external attribution but is already inherent in the *genesis* of the decisions.

[4] Cf. Thomae (1960) and, more recently, Damasio's (1994) theory of "somatic markers," i.e., bodily sensations such as the "gut feeling," which are necessary for successful decisions.

interpenetrate, so that the person becomes more transparent to herself and can identify with the choice. If successful, this process leads to the decision, the congruence experienced as evident: "That's how it is right for me."

The fact that we actually have the choice before making a decision is based on the suspension of previous impulses, on the space of possibility of thinking, and above all on our self-relationship. The decision then means an active "closing" of this space of possibility. But it can certainly not be understood as an act of an independent ego-instance, detached from the process of consideration, which at some point arbitrarily intervenes in the course of events. Rather, we must understand the entire movement of considering and deciding as a dynamic and open process, as a *life movement* in which the person making the decision is involved and always becomes "an other." Decisions are all the freer, the more aspects and deeper layers of the person enter into the dynamic process of consideration and feeling, the more transparent and at the same time perceptible the person becomes for himself. We are, as Bergson wrote, free "when our acts spring from our whole personality, when they express it" (Bergson 1910: 172).

The process thus involves a hermeneutic circle: the personal subject is not independent of it, but articulates, experiences itself, and develops within it. At the same time, however, it is also the overarching instance that drives and guides the process. In deliberating I do not move abstract possibilities back and forth idly but am constantly aware that I have to make the decision and that it depends on me, since it does not happen by itself. The decision is therefore only the culmination of a process that is both volitional and self-reflexive from the very beginning.

The choice of an alternative in the decision therefore does not itself have a higher-level reason outside the process to which it could be attributed. On the other hand, apart from indifferent, completely equivalent alternatives, it does not happen in an arbitrary or purely decisionistic way but *by the person identifying with an alternative*, taking it, and thus making the reasons corresponding to it effective. The self-relationship leads to the person's agreement with the choice and thus with the future which they assume for themself through their identification. The decision is therefore also experienced as self-fulfillment—and for this reason alone (and not because of a later social attribution) we experience ourselves as responsible for our actions.

If we summarize this analysis of the decision-making process, we can also define freedom of will as the ability of persons;

- to suspend their primary impulses;
- in a phase of moratorium, to form their own will according to their motives, convictions, and considerations;

- in the light of their self-relationship, to tentatively identify with the available possibilities;
- to achieve internal coherence or consistency in making the decision, and finally;
- to convert their decision into an action.

The triggering of action, which is the main focus of neurobiology, is thus only the last phase of the entire arc of a free action, which began with the suspension and interruption of the unproblematic way of life.

Embodied Freedom

So much for a brief phenomenology of decision making. How can we relate this representation to physiological processes in the brain and the body? The concept of embodied freedom ascribes decision neither to an immaterial mind nor to the brain. To decide and to act according to it means, as already mentioned, a self-determination that can only belong to the organism as a whole or to the living person. Therefore, if we want to develop a view of physiological processes that is compatible with an embodied freedom, we must revise the concept of so-called "mental causation" (Robb & Heil 2003). This is because it seems to imply that the mind intervenes in physiological processes, and thus gets into dualistic aporias. Instead, we need a causal approach that can be ascribed to the organism itself, and this consists in the *circular causality* of living beings.[5]

This term firstly describes the interrelation between the whole and the parts of a living system. A living being can be regarded as a self-organizing (autopoietic) system that continuously reproduces the components of which it is composed (organs, cells, macromolecules), while conversely these components constitute and maintain the system as a whole (Varela 1997). The whole is thus the condition of its parts, but it is also realized by them. Circular causality now means that the organism structures its components and integrates them into superordinate functions (*top down* or *downward causality*); at the same time, the components themselves act together in such a way that the overarching processes emerge (*bottom-up* or *upward causality*).

Such a circular causality characterizes, for instance, the relationship between genes and organism: the genetic structure of the individual cell nucleus controls the construction of specialized cell organs and functions (upward causality). Conversely, however, the configuration and functions of the entire organism

---

[5] The term comes from the "Synergetics" of Hermann Haken (2004); for detailed accounts see also Thompson 2007: 417ff.; Fuchs 2018: 94–100; and Fuchs 2020.

determine which genes are relevant for the development and regulation of a particular individual cell, for example, whether it develops into a muscle or a nerve cell (downward causality). Another example is physical activity such as walking: a variety of muscles, agonists, and antagonists must be integrated by the organism into a coordinated movement process, which they in turn also make possible.

Circular causality does not mean the appearance of new natural forces that contradict the laws of physics. Rather, macro-structures are in a position to *select* certain properties of their components and to *block* others through their form and configuration (Moreno & Umerez 2000). These components thus acquire new, emergent qualities: for example, iron embedded in hemoglobin is able to *reversibly* bind oxygen from the air we breathe, i.e., to release it again at a suitable point in the organism—while inorganic iron irreversibly rusts; it is unable to dissociate from oxygen again once the compound has formed. For such emergent properties no physical miracle is required but only a higher-order structure (in this case hemoglobin) which integrates its own structural elements into specific patterns of behavior. One can also understand downward causality in terms of Aristotelian *causa formalis*.

In this way, the processes of consciousness can also have a formative effect as superordinate structures in the physical behavior of the living being. Of course, the mental does not act as an external force upon brain or bodily processes but as a formative principle *in and through them*. When I speak, for example, the muscles of my tongue and larynx show certain ordered patterns of movement. Their direct efficient cause (*causa efficiens*) is the neuronally triggered release of acetylcholine at the motor end plates of the muscle fibers. However, it is also true to say that my tongue and larynx move in the same way *because I speak certain words* and focus on their intentional content. The primary, formative, or organizing cause of the muscle actions is my speaking (downward), which in turn is realized (upward) by a series of physiological mechanisms.

But the same is true for the *neuronal* processes in the motor or other areas of my brain that are necessary for this: they run in this particular way *because I speak these words*; there is no superordinate center in the brain that could produce or control this speech. Each neuronal subsystem and process, like the tongue and larynx, is only a necessary but not sufficient condition for the realization of my speech—the sufficient condition is nothing else but the living organism with its muscles, tendons, nerves, and neural networks *that I am*. The complete cause of my speech is therefore neither my tongue nor my brain (even if both are necessary to realize it) but I am this cause myself. In every conscious activity (speaking, writing, walking, thinking) the living person herself acts as the integral cause of the activity. As embodied processes of life, conscious processes can therefore be effective in the behavior of a person without influencing brain processes "from the outside."

Thus, we can now understand free decision-making and action as the self-steering of the organism, not on the basis of an interactionism between the mental and the physical, but of circular causality. Free decisions and actions are part of the overarching life process, which encompasses conscious deliberations and their corresponding neural activities as two different aspects. It is not least the phylogenetic and ontogenetic development of the brain that allows the human organism these degrees of freedom. This includes, in particular, prefrontal brain functions, which enable us to inhibit emotional impulses, but also to relativize the primarily dominant egocentric perspective in favor of another perspective and thus to become a morally responsible agent. The child acquires these abilities of self-control in the course of its social development, and they are also anchored in its brain in the course of these intersubjective experiences (Fuchs 2018: 202 ff.). The brain thus becomes indeed the organ of freedom—but only its organ, not its subject.

Counter Positions

With this, I have given a presentation and justification of the phenomenon of freedom of will from an embodied, libertarian point of view. Could this phenomenon still turn out to be an illusion? Let us consider the arguments for such an assumption. These fall essentially into two types:

1) External (scientifically based) objections: the world as a whole, or at least our brain, has a deterministic constitution, i.e., it is not set up in such a way that it allows freedom at all.

2) Immanent (philosophically based) objections: the idea of freedom as outlined here is essentially contradictory and therefore unsustainable.

Today, the strong or libertarian concept of freedom is usually contrasted with a *compatibilist* position according to which a restricted concept of freedom is consistent with determinism. I present this position following the external objections.

External Objections

Objections of this kind invoke either a general or a special (neurobiological) determinism.

General Determinism

Determinism is the metaphysical doctrine according to which the course of every event in the world is completely determined by initial conditions and laws of nature, so that there is only one possible future at any given time. In reference to Laplace's demon, one also speaks of Laplace determinism: a superior intelligence could, with complete knowledge of the state of the world at a given point in time, pre-calculate every future condition. Together with the assumption that the corresponding laws are physical laws, this results in *physicalism*: all events, including human actions, can in principle be fully explained in physical terms. The problem is obvious: if universal determinism were true, then there would be no more branching points in the course of the world and at no time would there be any more than *one* real possibility. But this makes the concept of decision pointless, because every idea of alternative possibilities we could have would have no influence on the course of the world.

There is a fundamental objection to this. To fix the course of the world as necessary and inevitable, the laws of nature would have to steer it in a certain direction, i.e., be able to *rule* it. To date, however, no law of nature has ever been presented that could make universally valid statements about the course of certain events, i.e., that would contain "always if, then" propositions about actual processes (Cartwright 1980; Keil 2007). When an apple falls to earth, Newton's law applies, but because of the superposition of other forces, it sometimes falls a little faster, sometimes a little slower; perhaps it does not reach the earth, but is caught by a bird before it does, and so on. So something can always happen in between. The actual course of the world is typified by overlaps, singularities, and chaotic processes. Moreover, probabilistic quantum physics has dealt a severe blow to the doctrine of universal determination.

Physicists generally admit that natural laws in their pure form only make statements about ideal objects in an ideal world (a world of models, in other words), whereas applied to the empirical world they are only valid approximately or *ceteris paribus*. This shows that laws of nature do not prescribe a world course without alternatives. According to more recent interpretations, they can only be understood as probabilistic regularities that describe in systematic form what happens or can happen. They therefore have no *prescriptive* but only *descriptive* validity (Cartwright 1997; Keil 2007).

The scientific-theoretical status of natural laws has therefore changed considerably. The divinely decreed "force of law," which was still attributed to them in the eighteenth century, has been replaced by the more modest status of regularities which observable natural processes exhibit. The lawfulness that we observe in these processes is based on what is actually happening in the world, not the other way round. Of course, natural laws exclude certain possibilities and are therefore restrictive; but if they are satisfied, room for maneuver always remains. To give an example, the laws of nature exclude the possibility of me jumping into orbit, but they do not determine where I will travel to on my next vacation. Laplace's determinism would, however, require that there be an arrangement of the world that excludes all but one possibility. Such lawful arrangements with causal force do not exist in physics. But, if we do not find in respect to certain courses of events any laws which are always valid, and allow infallible prediction, then the claim that there must be such laws and that our knowledge of them has simply not progressed far enough becomes an article of faith. Such events would include, in particular, human actions.

Specific Determinism

Does determinism then apply at least to specific areas, for example to processes in the human brain? Contrary to what neuroscientists often suggest, there are in fact no deterministic neurobiological laws that would even allow the prediction of a certain person's actions in the next few seconds or minutes. Good psychological knowledge is far better suited to this. This is not only due to the complexity of the brain but also to its dependence on the individual's previous history; above all it is due to the brain's plasticity and constant remodeling during every interaction with the environment. Under these conditions, it would be a pointless undertaking to search for deterministic laws for the activities of the brain or the actions of a person. Even Libet and his successors, whose experiments on freedom of will deal with a timeframe of mere seconds, can at best calculate statistical probabilities for the occurrence of subsequent actions from observing brain processes.[6] But, regardless of whether the probability is 30, 50, 70, or 95 percent—it would still not be sufficient to prove a determinism of the brain. There is no such thing as "a bit of determinism"—either it applies completely or not at all.

Of course, correlations between experience or action and brain processes do not prove determinism either. They are usually expressed in formulations according to which brain processes "underlie" actions, "realize" them, "control," or "trigger" them, and so on. Such vocabulary, however, while giving a deterministic impression, does not imply a strict determination by natural law. Looking more closely, neurobiologists merely claim, but do not prove, the determinism of the brain. Empirical evidence rather points to the contrary: contingencies can be found in abundance on the molecular and cellular level of the brain: fluctuations of the membrane potential through opening and closing of ion channels, the release of transmitter packages or the activation of individual neurons are non-deterministic and cannot be predicted exactly (Falkenburg 2012: 295 ff.). This randomness is not necessarily blurred at higher levels but

---

[6] See, for example, the more recent experiments on free will by John-Dylan Haynes (Soon et al. 2008).

can even be enhanced by appropriate adjustment of the system's non-linearities and propagated to macroscopic levels (Braun 2021).

Let me summarize. Anyone who believes that freedom of choice is incompatible with the scientific view of the world or is compatible only if the concept of freedom is adapted and subordinated in advance to the postulated determinism (see the following section), is misjudging the scientific situation. This supposed "scientific world view" has little to do with the practice of natural science. Rather, one can speak of a *scientistic* view of the world, which of course is not empirically based but has the character of a metaphysical doctrine. I maintain that we do not find any empirical findings in the scientific world that are insurmountably opposed to our experience of freedom of choice.

The Compatibilist Counter Position

Let us now look at the currently most frequently held counter position to the libertarian concept of freedom, namely compatibilism: according to this, freedom and determination of the will are compatible. The price of this theory is high, however: the weaker freedom which, according to compatibilists, is supposed to satisfy us is essentially only the *freedom of action*, i.e., the ability to act according to our wishes, free from external or internal compulsion. What the compatibilist must deny is the *freedom of choice*, i.e., the ability to decide differently when facing alternatives.

Admittedly, the intuitions we have against compatibility are serious. Whoever hears for the first time of the view that the will is at the same time free and strictly determined will find this absurd. How can our sense of responsibility be reconciled with an inevitable course of action, with our inability to do anything else? Compatibilists usually try nevertheless to rescue a sense of speaking of alternative possibilities, namely by saying: "A person *could* have acted differently if she had decided differently," which implies: "Since she did not decide differently, she could not have acted differently either." This is a cunning linguistic-philosophical reinterpretation, but the objection is obvious: how could the person have decided differently, if she was determined to do so? Bieri therefore goes back a step further: Raskolnikov could have decided differently if he had *thought* differently (2001: 322). But how could he have thought differently? To do so, the course of the world would have had to branch *even earlier*, but that too would have been ruled out by determinism. Every choice we make would already have been predetermined by earlier events outside our sphere of influence.

This means: the actual ability to act differently is not to be grasped by a fictitious variation of the circumstances of a decision but is itself *a special state of open possibility* in which the individual finds himself. When I ask myself whether I will accept an attractive job offer or keep my secure position, from a libertarian point of view the decision is *actually* not yet fixed; I could still do *both* A *and* B. The compatibilist, on the other hand, circumvents this real possibility of alternatives by *only fictitiously changing* what is really given, just to be able to say that under these fictitious circumstances another course of action would have been possible. However, this is not entirely fair. For the hypothetically assumed alternative course of events—I could have "thought differently"—could only have become reality if I had been a different person, indeed if *the course of the world as a whole* had been different. In the end, however, this means nothing other than that I *could not* act differently at all.

Similar to Bieri, Pauen & Roth (2008) have proposed an interpretation of alternative possibilities that attempts to delineate a separate area in universal determinism, so to speak, namely the self-determination of a person. According to this interpretation, an action is self-determined if it can be traced back to the persons themselves, or more precisely to their personal preferences, convictions, and desires, that they carry out action A and not an alternative B. The conformity of the decision and action with one's own preferences is a sufficient characteristic of free decisions, even if these existing preferences in turn determine the result. This would also satisfy general determinism, because even if the action can ultimately be traced back to physically determined neuronal processes, it is precisely those processes that also underlie the preferences of the person (Pauen & Roth 2008: 39, 42).

Can we be reassured by the fact that we can, in a sense, attribute our own branch of events to ourselves in the universal context of determination? This is only possible if this branch is itself subject to our own possible influence. Pauen & Roth (2008: 55) therefore emphasize that personal preferences can in principle become the objects of effective decisions: I could come to the decision to abandon my conviction of the illegality of stealing, since I attribute it only to my conventional upbringing, and accordingly decide freely to steal in future.

But this again shifts the problem of being able to act differently into the past: how should I be able to ascribe to myself a conviction as freely chosen when the determinants of this choice have in turn escaped my influence? The fact that I am able to critically reflect on my preferences, convictions, and character traits when adopted by others does not change my lack of freedom toward them, as long as their alteration is either random or deterministic. The presumed freedom of choice leads to an ultimately deterministic view of the self. The freedom of differential action is not saved from determinism by recourse to personal preferences if the freedom of being able *to be different* cannot be made plausible. It remains the case that the universal deterministic causal connection makes the concept of alternative possibilities meaningless.

I will not go into further detail on the compatibilist position, but I will conclude by discussing some of the objections often raised against the libertarian position and which try to prove it to be self-contradictory. In my responses, I will draw in particular on arguments of Robert Kane (1996) and Geert Keil (2007).

Immanent Objections

(1) *Objection of dualism.* Does libertarian freedom imply, as is often assumed by its opponents, that an immaterial mind influences the body world when we make decisions?

No, the libertarian point of view does not presuppose dualistic interaction. Conscious experiences are embodied, i.e., physically realized, but this does not mean that they have to be physically determined. The concept of embodied freedom, as advocated here, implies that we are only free as embodied subjects, i.e., that consciousness can only perform a controlling and effective function when it is embedded in the organism and carried by physical processes. There can be no interaction at all between an activity of consciousness and the neuronal substrate processes, neither a causality in one direction nor in the other—especially not once both are seen as moments of a unified conduct of life, as functions of the organism, which only appear to us under different aspects.[7] The fact that there are neuronal correlations of conscious events does not endanger our freedom, on the contrary—provided that no additional neuro-deterministic assumption comes into play (Keil 2007: 96).

(2) *Objection of the causal gap.* Does libertarian freedom presuppose local gaps of indeterminism in the otherwise deterministic course of the Universe? Are we freed, for example, by quantum leaps that give the will the indeterminacy it needs, and from which it could, as it were, begin?

No, because non-determinacy is not an exceptional event but a global constitution of the world—there are no deterministic laws for the actual course of the world. No event is Laplace-determined in the sense that it has been fixed from the very beginning of the universe. Of course, what is predicted often happens, but even more often it is impossible to predict what will happen; and everything that is not impossible in terms of natural laws remains possible. In what way such a non-determined state can be defined more precisely in the brain remains an open question—it may be that quantum-physical indeterminacies in connection with chaos theory play a role here. For the time being it is sufficient to

---

[7] See Fuchs 2018, 2020 on this fundamental concept.

reject the claim that all neuronal events were strictly determined—it is simply not proven.

A causal gap would also not appear in any detailed naturalistic description of human actions. To illustrate this, we can imagine that a fictitious physicist is able to describe all the actions that I will perform in the course of the day wholly in terms of movements of matter, to calculate the masses, forces, and fields involved and to relate them to physical laws. None of my actions will violate the laws of nature and yet it would be absurd to believe that the whole sequence of states of my organism could be explained or even predicted by the means of physics. The level of human deliberations, reasons, motives, and intentions simply does not appear in the calculations; likewise, their effectiveness remains *physically* unobservable. In order to secure our experience of freedom we therefore only need to assume that the neuronal carrier processes are *not exclusively* determined by physical laws, or in other words, that my actions are *physically underdetermined*. The causal principle—every event has a cause— remains valid, but it does not imply determinism. The superior and complete cause of a free action, however, is the embodied person themself, not certain events in their body.

(3) *Objection of the absolute will.* A frequent objection to the libertarian concept of freedom is that a will that is free in the strong sense must be a quasi-absolute will that is not conditioned by anything, and must be independent of the attitudes, wishes, and preferences of the willing person (Bieri 2001). Such a will would then only happen to us and we would not be able to attribute it to ourselves. We could rightly refuse to accept any responsibility for such a will that would come over us like a *deus ex machina*. All this sounds convincing. The problem is that no representative of libertarian freedom has ever posited such an absolute will, and it is not even necessary. For even if we are free to choose between alternative possibilities, the alternatives remain meaningfully linked to our abilities, inclinations and deliberations. The will can be conditional and still free. This becomes even clearer in the following.

(4) *Objection of arbitrariness.* Closely linked to the last one is probably the most common objection to the libertarian view: a completely free decision between two justified alternatives must ultimately be an unfounded one, because the reasons for deciding should not have any causal force to bring about the decision. The person could then choose both A and B *under the same conditions and for the same reasons*. This would mean that the decision would not be the result of the previous deliberation but of pure coincidence or mere arbitrariness. But we cannot attribute a random or irrational action to ourselves or to others since no one would then be responsible for it. It seems as if we are actually getting into an aporia here: either an action happens with unavoidable

necessity or by chance and irrational arbitrariness, and both are incompatible with our intuition of freedom.

This has to be countered as follows: the openness of the decision-making process does not mean that a person who, having deliberated, concludes that A is preferable to B, could still just as well do B—that would indeed be irrational. After having clarified the alternatives and having committed oneself to one of them, to be able just as well to do the opposite—that would not be what is required with the freedom of choice between alternative possibilities. Rather, the whole decision-making process, as shown previously, is to be seen as a temporal unity, as a life movement. This means that the state of the person at time t_1 is, in a certain sense, included in their later states t_2, t_3, t_4, etc.; in other words, none of these states exist in isolation or "in cross section." The state immediately before the decision integrates the whole course of the decision process.[8] Its openness does not mean that the space of possibility remains unchanged in the course of the process, that thinking about it starts again from zero every time.

But the person could still hesitate at the end of their deliberations, they could suspend their decision again and reconsider. Then the process might lead to outcome B instead of outcome A. But even then, the person will carry out action B for understandable reasons—they just had good reasons for A *as well as* for B (Kane (1996: 126) speaks of a "two-way rationality"). Hence, to act differently under given circumstances does not mean irrational arbitrariness, as if our will happened to us out of nowhere—it means rather that there is always the possibility of renewed suspension and thus of "thinking things over" (see also Keil 2007: 114). If the person finally ends this process—for whatever reason, be it because they are under pressure of time or because a choice seems sufficiently coherent to them—*it is they who make the reason in question effective by completing the process.* Because reasons as such only make us inclined, but do not force us. And there is no higher-level reason that causes us to prefer the reasons for A to those for B. In a decision, therefore, a volitional, sometimes even decisionistic element comes into play. But this does not make the decision blind or irrational, because there were good reasons for both A and B, and these reasons ensure that the person is able in both cases to make their actions their own.

Now this consideration seems to come very close to the compatibilist reinterpretation: "If person P had thought and decided differently, he would also have acted differently." Indeed, the libertarian will not dispute this retrospective

---

[8] A precondition for this integration can be seen in Husserl's analysis of inner time consciousness: every present moment still contains the *retentions* of the preceding moments, albeit (looking into the past) in an increasingly attenuated or superimposed form (Husserl 1991).

formulation; he will only interpret it differently, namely not as a hypothetical variation in another world, but as a factual statement about the decision-making process. The libertarian insists that the fundamental indeterminacy and openness of one's own future enables the person to make a decision in this or that way under the *given* conditions.[9] Being able to think and decide differently is then no longer fictional but accompanies the decision-making process as a real "alternativity." Unlike the determinist, the libertarian does not have to change the pre-history of the actual action or fictitiously assume that the actor has a different personality with different preferences in order to speak legitimately of *being able to do things differently under the given circumstances.*

Conclusion

My starting point was our libertarian intuition of the practical reality of our experience of freedom. This experience is undeniable, and determinisms based on natural science or psychology can, in a sense, only sow secondary and external doubts about this reality. The compatibilist attempt at compromise, by contrast—the assumption that a strict terminology is compatible with a reduced concept of freedom—is reminiscent of Orwell's "doublethink," which allows the philosopher or natural scientist to maintain a closed physical world view on the one hand and to continue to live in everyday life according to our intuition of freedom on the other.

This clear life-worldly intuition justifies distributing the burden of proof to the disadvantage of the deterministic position. Anyone who denies freedom in the strong sense needs very convincing arguments for doing so; general deterministic postulates or questionably interpreted empirical research findings are not enough. I have tried to show that there are no convincing objections to our libertarian intuition. But it is due to the dominance of scientific and scientistic thinking in our culture that the burden of proof has now almost reversed. Freedom today finds itself in a position where it has to justify itself; indeed, it seems to be becoming an anachronism that only a few unenlightened or backward-looking individuals seriously cling to. This is encouraged by the ever-expanding doctrine of the *Grand Illusion*, according to which our primary life-world experience can only have an illusory and virtual character in a physical world. Of course, we know that even if freedom turned out to be only an illusion, this illusion would not disappear in practice. And that is precisely why

---

[9] It is obvious that the *retrospective* deliberation still retains a hypothetical character: of course, it cannot change the past decision. But it is nevertheless valid insofar as it projects the assumption of a person's present freedom of choice back into the past.

deterministic positions can also be advocated with a certain frivolity. If freedom does not exist, then let us simply pretend it does—why not?

It may be that this attitude corresponds to a tendency that will prevail in the end. But I would like to offer one last thing for consideration: if we accept the framework of determinism for our lives, this would not only have consequences for our sense of responsibility and the social institutions based on it, such as criminal law. Above all, it would mean that we would no longer think our lives and our world in terms of an open future; that we would have less appreciation of the possibility of the new, the creative in the world, and instead lock ourselves in the cage of universal determinism. The future would no longer be an open space of possibilities but would be iron-clad by past conditions and natural laws. To think and understand oneself as a being that obtains its possibilities of development from the future and that is able to grasp them in an ever new way—this seems to me to be the core of an image of the human that is worth standing up for.

References

Aristotle. 2002. *Nicomachean Ethics.* C. **Rowe** (trans.) Oxford: Oxford University Press.

Bergson, H. 1910. *Time and Free Will: An Essay on the Immediate Data of Consciousness.* F.L. Pogson (trans.). London: George Allen and Unwin. (First Published 1889.)

Bieri, P. 2001. *Das Handwerk der Freiheit: Über die Entdeckung des eigenen Willens.* München: Hanser.

Braun, H. A. 2021. Stochasticity versus determinacy in neurobiology: from ion channels to the question of the "free will". *Frontiers in Systems Neuroscience* 15: 39.

Cartwright, N. 1980. "Do the laws of physics state the facts?" *Pacific Philosophical Quarterly* **61**: 75–84.

Cartwright, N. 1997. "Models: The blueprints for laws." *Philosophy of Science* **64**: 292–303.

Damasio, A. 1994. *Descartes' Error: Emotion, Reason and the Human Brain.* New York: Avon Books.

Falkenburg, B. 2012. *Mythos Determinismus: Wieviel erklärt uns die Hirnforschung?* Berlin, Heidelberg: Springer.

Fuchs, T. 2018. *Ecology of the Brain. The Phenomenology and Biology of the Embodied Mind.* Oxford: Oxford University Press.

Fuchs, T. 2020. "The circularity of the embodied mind." *Frontiers in Psychology* **11**: 1707.

Haggard, P. 2011. "Decision time for free will." *Neuron* **69**: 404–406.

Haken, H. 2004. *Synergetics: Introduction and Advanced Topics.* Berlin, Heidelberg: Springer.

Husserl, E. 1991. *On the Phenomenology of the Consciousness of Internal Time.* **John Barnett Brough** (trans.) Dordrecht: Kluwer.

Kane, R. 1996. *The Significance of Free Will.* Oxford, New York: Oxford University Press.

Kant, I. 1999. "Review of Schulz's attempt at introduction to a doctrine of morals for all human beings regardless of different religions." In I. Kant (ed.), *Practical Philosophy*. Mary J. Gregor (trans.) Cambridge: Cambridge University Press. (First published 1783.)

Keil, G. 2007. *Willensfreiheit*. Berlin: De Gruyter.

Lindemann, G. 2007. "Plädoyer für einen methodologisch pluralistischen Monismus." In H.-P. Krüger (ed.) *Hirn als Subjekt? Philosophische Grenzfragen der Neurobiologie*. Berlin: Akademie-Verlag (pp. 401–410).

Libet, B. 1985. "Unconscious cerebral initiative and the role of conscious will in voluntary action." *Behavioral and Brain Sciences* 8: 529–566.

Locke, J. 1997. *An Essay Concerning Human Understanding*. London: Penguin. (Originally Published 1689.)

Moore, G. E. 1912. *Ethics*. London: Williams & Norgate.

Moreno, A., J. Umerez. 2000. "Downward causation at the core of living organization." In P. B. Andersen, C. Emmeche, N. O. Finnemann, P. V. Christiansen (eds.) *Downward Causation: Minds, Bodies and Matter*. Aarhus: Aarhus University Press (pp. 99–117).

Nida-Rümelin, J. 2005. *Über menschliche Freiheit*. Stuttgart: Reclam.

Pauen, M., G. Roth. 2008. *Freiheit, Schuld und Verantwortung: Grundzüge einer naturalistischen Theorie der Willensfreiheit*. Frankfurt/M.: Suhrkamp.

Robb, D., J. Heil. 2003. Mental causation. *Stanford Encyclopedia of Philosophy*. E. N. Zalta (ed.), https://plato.stanford.edu/archives/sum2019/entries/mental-causation/>.

Soon, C. S., M. Brass, H. J. Heinze, J. D. Haynes. 2008. "Unconscious determinants of free decisions in the human brain." *Nature Neuroscience* 11(5): 543–545.

Swaab, D. F. 2014. *We Are Our Brains: A Neurobiography of the Brain, From the Womb to Alzheimer's*. London: Penguin.

Thomae, H. 1960. *Der Mensch in der Entscheidung*. München: Barth.

Thompson, E. 2007. *Mind in Life: Biology, Phenomenology, and the Sciences of Mind*. Cambridge/MA: Harvard University Press.

Varela, F. J. 1997. "Patterns of life: Intertwining identity and cognition." *Brain and Cognition* 34: 72–87.

Chapter 6

Brain World or Life World?
Critique of Neuroconstructivism

Introduction

That everything people experience is in reality a construction and simulation of their brains is one of the common beliefs of neuroscientists and neuro-philosophers today. From pain or anger to colors or music, to love or faith, there is hardly a phenomenon that is not accommodated somewhere in the brain. The cosmos is created in the head, and perception becomes a physiological illusion, so to speak. Typical descriptions run as follows:

> What you see is not what is really there, it is what your brain believes is there. (Crick 1994: 31)

> Multimedia mind-show occurs constantly as the brain processes external and internal sensory events. (Damasio 1999: 112)

> [W]e find ourselves always already in a biologically generated "Phenospace": within a virtual reality generated by mental simulation. (Metzinger 1999: 243; trans. T. F.)

So, this is the worldview of neuroconstructivism: we are enclosed in our brain like a mussel in its shell, and the qualitative world of the senses is a world of illusion.[1] The tree in front of me is actually not green, its flowers do not smell, the bird in its branches does not sing melodically: these are all just functional illusory worlds that the brain creates instead of naked, material-kinematic processes. It is impossible to say what the tree looks like in reality, because it "doesn't look like" at all—it consists only of abstract, mathematically describ-able particles, waves, and quantities. Indeed, our consciousness itself is only a simulation that the brain calculates from such physical particles and quantities, called information.

Now the neurobiological enterprise of naturalizing the mind is only the last step in a process of de-anthropomorphization, the splitting between the life-world and science, which goes back to the Early-Modern period. Already for

---

[1] Similar positions are also held by Swaab (2014), Eagleman (2015) or Seth (2021).

In Defense of the Human Being. Thomas Fuchs, Oxford University Press. © Suhrkamp Verlag 2021.
DOI: 10.1093/oso/9780192898197.003.0007

Galileo, Descartes, and other protagonists of the naturalization project, the world is not what it appears to us in everyday experience. Its actual nature is not accessible to perception; it first has to be revealed in mathematical terms. In this way, the living world acquires the illusory status described previously: we think, says Descartes, "that we see the torch itself and hear the bell, and not that we only feel the movements proceeding from them" (Descartes 1649/1989: 31). Perception only conveys *representations* of the things in our consciousness, that means, illusory images, conveniently generated by the organization of our natural senses. Only science can give us information about the world we actually live in.

Of course, Descartes' dualistic ontology has long been on the retreat today. Materialism solves the problem caused by the split between the perceived world and the scientifically conceived Universe by attributing ontological reality only to the latter. In one point, however, the advocates of modern naturalism still link up with Descartes and the idealism that followed him: for them, too, the perceived world is only a subjective phenomenon, namely a sequence of "representations" or "models" as inner representatives of the outer world. Neurobiology adopts this idealistic conception of perception, however fiercely it otherwise fights dualism. It is satisfied with materialistically reinterpreting the concept of representation, namely as designating those neuronal processes which are supposed to underlie the subjective images of the external world. Through specific excitation patterns or data structures, the brain reflects the structures of the environment. As it turns out, the idealistic inner world of consciousness and the neurobiological inner world of the brain fit together surprisingly well: because from both an idealistic and a materialistic point of view, the subject has no real share in the world. The link between the two traditions is established by the epistemology of neuroconstructivism.

Now, there is an area of the world that resists banishment to an inner mental world in a special way: it is *our own body* that we inhabit, not like captains inhabit their ships or drivers their cars, but in the way that *we ourselves are this body*—in the felt spatial extension and mineness of bodily sensations, in the felt mobility of the limbs and in all bodily abilities through which we deal with the world. The body is the primary medium of being in the world, and thus also the center of our life-world. The program of naturalization can therefore only be carried out consistently if it is possible to prove this subjective body as an illusion or projection and to put the physically defined body in its place. It is no coincidence that Descartes already invested considerable effort in undermining the primary spatiality and mineness of the experienced body. Above all, phenomena such as the phantom limb, which amputes feel in the place of the missing limb, but also the arbitrary divisibility of the body in contrast to the mind, were intended to convince his contemporaries that the old, Aristotelian-Thomist conception of the *coextension* of soul and body was to be abandoned (Descartes 1641/2008: 61 ff.). The soul is located in the brain, more precisely in the pineal gland, not in the body as a whole. The close connection, indeed merging of soul and body, which Descartes nevertheless conceded (ibid.: 57), should not change the fact that the soul does not need the body conglomerate and is radically different from it.

We encounter the same problem today in neuroconstructivism, albeit under materialistic auspices. In the interest of the naturalization program, bodily subjectivity must be proved to be only a construct. The phantom limb and related experiences in healthy people, in which bodily sensations are localized outside the body limits, even the so-called out-of-body experiences are taken to prove that our subjective body is nothing more than a *habitual phantom body*, a simulation or construction of the brain, which under certain circumstances can be created at almost any point in space. For example, the brain researcher Ramachandran lists two experiments that can be easily carried out by anyone on spatial displacements of bodily experience outside the body.[2] These are intended to prove:

> Your own [subjective] body is a phantom, one that your brain has temporarily constructed purely for convenience. (Ramachandran & Blakeslee 1998: 58)

The spatial body schema, proprioception, the sensations of movement or kinesthesia—all of these are thus generated at certain brain areas, primarily the parietal cortex, and projected into the virtual space constructed by the brain. The result is a *split between the organic body and the subjective body*, as if these belonged to two different worlds—one to the physical world and the other to a virtual "inner world" of consciousness produced by the brain. This would apply to all bodily sensations:

> Pain itself is an illusion – constructed entirely in your brain like any other sensory experience. (Ramachandran & Blakeslee 1998: 58)

---

[2] One of the best-known experiments of this kind is the "rubber hand illusion": If a visible rubber hand on the table is rhythmically touched synchronously with the subject's own hand hidden under the table, the subject will gradually come to feel the rubber hand as his or her own hand actually being "touched" (Botvinick & Cohen 1998). Metzinger and Blanke have extended this principle to a whole-body illusion: if a test person uses video glasses to create the perception of a virtual body outside themselves, and the back of this virtual body is now stroked at the same time as their own back, it results in a shift of self-awareness into the virtual body (Blanke & Metzinger 2008).

> You can reach out and touch the material of the physical world [...] But this sense of touch is not a direct experience. Although it feels like the touch is happening in your fingers, in fact it's all happening in the mission control center of the brain. It's the same across all your sensory experiences [...] your brain has never directly experienced the external world, and it never will. (Eagleman 2015: 40 f.)

Now, certainly the brain has never experienced the external world, since it cannot in principle experience anything. But what about myself? Is my spatial sense of touch in my fingers or pain in my foot only an illusion? If perception is to convey more than a virtual world, and if the life-world is to be restored to its rightful place against the neuroscientific claim to dominance, then obviously the asserted virtuality of bodily experience must be refuted. In the following I will develop an argumentation for this, which is based on the implicit intersubjectivity of perception. As we will see, it is capable of authenticating our experience of existing bodily in the world and thus refuting the idea of a monadic inner world in the brain.

Bodily Being-in-the-World: The Coextension of Lived Body and Physical Body

Let us first envision the fact that we normally experience the subjective or lived body (*Leib*) and the organic body (*Körper*) as *coextensive*. The potter feels the clay exactly where his or her hand, in fact, presses and forms it. The pain felt is located where the needle pierces the physical body. Indeed, if the patient shows the doctor his painful foot, the latter will also look there for a cause. If the subjective experience of the lived body were only an illusion, the doctor could ignore the patient's statement and, instead of that, examine his brain. There is thus a spatial correspondence or *syntopy* between the lived body and the physical body. Although the phenomenon of phantom pain shows us the exceptional case that the organism can also produce a sensation of pain without the respective limb, this does not make the normal case any less astonishing. How is it actually possible that we feel the pain where the matching wounded part of the body is situated too, and not, for example, in the brain?

The obvious assumption of a "projection" of bodily sensations into the space of the body does not lead us any further, because in a virtual subjective world this objective body space would not exist at all. There cannot be a projection "toward the outside" if this outside is, according to the assumption, merely an interior world constructed by the brain. The notion of projection, which was once rather commonplace, has thus largely been replaced in the cognitive neurosciences by a unified virtual-phenomenal space, or a "phenospace" (Metzinger 2009: 221). Consequently, then, the perceived prick of the needle, which causes the pain, must also be declared a virtual construct or a simulation of the brain, as well as the foot I see before me and with it the whole environment I perceive. We would then have absolutely no access to actual reality.

However, as soon as we enter an *intersubjective* situation, such as the patient already mentioned visiting a doctor, it becomes immediately clear that the subjective experience and the objective situation, the sensation of pain and its observable physical cause, in no way belong to two separate worlds. The syntopy or the coincidence of the place of pain and injury now involves the body perceived by *both* the doctor and the patient. Just there where the patient feels the pain and where he points to is where the doctor also finds its cause. Both see the same foot which subjectively hurts *and* is objectively injured. How is this possible?

Here, we first have to show that a reference to the respective "phenospaces" of doctor and patient no longer makes sense—if talk about a reality of the body is meaningful at all, then it is so in the intersubjective situation, because, in this context, the subjective spaces of both persons coincide in a way which *cancels their mere subjectivity*. The argument goes as follows.

Since, according to the neuroconstructivist premise, every brain only produces its own virtual space, there cannot be any "shared phenospace" of doctor and patient. Because if perception could, without remainder, be described and explained as a physical process happening between an object and a brain, then *two persons could never observe one and the same object*. The two processes would run, starting from the object, in different directions and remain strictly separated from one another. Both persons would thus be locked in their particular worlds, all the more so since they remain mere simulations for each other—in the end leading to a *neuro-solipsism*.

But even the simple process of the doctor writing a prescription for a painkiller and handing the paper over to the patient rests on the fact that both see and handle the same object, and not just deal with their own internal constructs or images. Both have a share in the intersubjectively constituted, and thus objective space of a common world. Their subjective view is, admittedly, an individual, perspectival view. However, it is not "only subjective" in the sense that what is seen is merely virtual or "in the subject." In seeing, we always already find ourselves in a common space with other sighted people (whether they are present or absent), whose perspectives we assume to be equally valid. It is their seeing (or hearing, touching, etc.,) that authenticates our own perception. The intentionality of perception thus removes the attachment to a purely subjective perspective; it contains an *implicit intersubjectivity*.[3]

---

[3] This will be discussed in more detail in chapter 7. According to Husserl, it is precisely the horizon-like nature of given objects that testifies to the fact that they are also accessible to

Doctor and patient therefore perceive the same, objective body. Now, the subjective place of the patient's pain concurs with the objective place of the body part. Hence, the subjective-bodily and the objective space *in reality* coincide and we must repeat the question: how is it possible that the patient feels the pain *there* and not, for example, in the brain?

The form of the question admittedly shows that we in the Cartesian tradition are still used to categorically separating subjectivity from the living organism. Things are completely different, though, once we think in evolutionary terms: originally the whole body was, in certain ways, a sensing and feeling organ. Precisely at its surfaces which border on the environment, the organism is irritable, sensitive, and responsive. *Elementary sensitivity begins at the periphery of the body.* The development of a central nervous system does not remove peripheral sensitivity but integrates it by means of a peripheral nervous system spread over the whole body. The fact that bodily consciousness still remains coextensive with the organism shows that it does not spring out of it as a separate entity, like Athena from the head of Zeus, but is, from the very beginning, an *embodied and extended* consciousness. It represents the *"integral"*[4] *of the living organism as a whole*, not a phenomenon encapsulated in the brain.

Seen in this way, the coextension of the subjective, lived body and the material organic body is no longer surprising. It is, however, functionally meaningful too: conscious experience is where our interactions with the environment take place—in the periphery, not in the brain. After all, the body is the actual "player on the field." That is why it is meaningful that its borders, positions and movements in the environment are experienced in "analog" form, i.e., in the space of the lived body, not only cognitively registered.

Theoretically, it would also be conceivable that pains would become conscious in a placeless manner, like thoughts or memories. However, without the coincidence of the two spaces, we would only have our body as an external, pliable tool and would not be "incarnated" in it. Only because consciousness is in the painful hand is it withdrawn involuntarily from the pricking needle.

....

others: the object of experience, for example a table, is not exhausted in the aspects given to me, but has a horizon of simultaneous aspects (such as the back of the table) which can in principle be perceived by others. Because of its aspectuality, the object does not only exist for me alone, but always refers to others at the same time (Husserl 1962: 468). Thus, my aching foot is also a foot implicitly seen by others.

4 In algebra, the integral enables the calculation of an area that is bounded by a function over a certain basis. I use it as a metaphor to signify the integration which consciousness achieves over an extended basis, without being separable from that basis as a "representation." Even if the brain is the *conditio sine qua non* for this integration, it does not become the "seat" of consciousness.

Only because the feeling of the potter is in the touching hand by which they feel the clay can they also mold it skillfully. A mere "central processing" in the brain could never achieve what the immediate presence of the subject in his or her hand makes possible, that is the linking of perception, movement, and objects into a common, intermodal action space: "My body is wherever there is something to be done" (Merleau-Ponty 1962: 224).

Therefore, if I grasp for something, I move *and I feel* not a virtual but a real hand which, for its part, touches a real object. That becomes possible by the fact that the subjective bodily space is embedded in the objective space of the organism in its environment. This means we are actually in the world as bodily beings (*leibhaftig*)—we are not beings who only have the illusory feeling of inhabiting our bodies.

Admittedly, the extension of the subjective, lived body is flexible—that is, according to the particular functional requirements. It does not always square exactly with the limits of the physical body. That is why instruments can also be integrated in the subjective body schema. When using a walking stick, one does not feel the resistance of the surface in one's hand, but at the tip of the stick.[5] Likewise, the experienced driver can feel the quality of the road coating literally under the tires of his car, or the width of the garage walls through which the car still fits. A person who has had a limb amputated learns to "incorporate" his prosthesis by adapting to it, so that it becomes a new felt limb for him. In fact, even a rubber hand can temporarily connect to the felt body if it is included in the loops of sensation, perception and movement in a coordinated manner—in just the same way as in ventriloquism the speaker's disguised voice is attributed to a dummy. In all these cases, far from being "merely illusions," the optimal coherence of the various sensory and kinesthetic modalities is established within the intermodal action-perception space of the body.[6]

Instead of being only a central construct, the subjective space of the lived body is therefore modified depending on the particular border at which the *actual* interaction with the environment takes place. This is, in turn, functionally

---

[5] "The blind man's stick has ceased to be an object for him, and is no longer perceived for itself; its point has become an area of sensitivity, extending the scope and active radius of touch" (Merleau-Ponty 1962: 127).

[6] On the one hand, one may call the rubber hand experience an illusion—after all, one's hand is actually being touched under the table. "But in another sense there's no illusion – or rather, the mechanisms at work in this illusion, if we want to call it that, are those of normal, successful perception" (Noë 2009: 74). It is important to note that so-called illusions do not prove perception *as such* to be illusory or merely a "veridical hallucination"; on the contrary, they point to the synthetic or gestalt-forming activity of perceiving which renders the environment available and viable for a living and moving being.

meaningful: physical contact with the actual resistance of the surroundings must feed into the person's subjective experience, so that adequate handling of objects and tools is made possible. The supposed "illusions" which arise from this are, in reality, highly meaningful extensions of our subjective body schema in contact with the environment. This means that the objective space of the physical organism and the subjective space of bodily experience are intertwined and mutually modify one another.

However, one restriction applies: phenomena such as phantom limbs or phantom pains show that the discrepancy between the objective-bodily and the subjective-bodily space can, in exceptional cases, assume considerable proportions. Yet, just like the phenomena of extension in tool use mentioned previously, such exceptions do not contradict the *basic syntopy*, i.e., the coextensive spatiality of living and organic body—on the contrary, they even confirm it. If *Leib* and *Körper* were not normally coextensive, the amputee would not find his phantom limb so irritating, because there would not arise any *discrepancy* between both kinds of space.[7] Admittedly, the forms and boundaries of the sensed body are normally blurred and fluid; for this reason alone, they cannot correspond exactly to the physical body structures. However, only the fundamental syntopy is at stake here, if we want to refute the illusion thesis or the idea of a mere "phantom body." Just as the occurrence of optical illusions does not prove our visual perception as such to be an illusion, phantom limbs or out-of-body experiences do not allow the conclusion to be drawn that our bodily experience is generally virtual.

The Locus of Pain

In the light of these reflections, let us now ask again: where is the pain when my foot hurts me? According to common neuroscientific belief, it is where it is produced, that is, in the brain. Even John Searle, a prominent critic of neurobiological reductionism, is of this opinion:

> Common sense tells us that our pains are in physical space within our bodies, that for example, a pain in the foot is literally inside the area of the foot. But we now know that is false. The brain forms a body image, and pains, like all bodily sensations, are parts of the body image. The pain-in-the-foot is literally in the physical space of the brain. (Searle 1992: 63)

---

[7] Thus, an arm amputee can move his stump toward a wall and, to his dismay, notice how the phantom effortlessly penetrates the wall and now occupies "the same" space with it (cf. Katz 1921). But, neither of the two experienced spaces is illusionary in itself—they are rather coextensive, overlapping modalities of the unified experiential space.

However, the brain neither feels nor contains pain. It does not produce a "body image" either, for the experienced body is not an image of a body, it is rather the body itself *as felt*. The only thing that can be found in the brain when somebody feels pain are neuronal activations in the somatosensory cortex and in the cingulate gyrus, and however much these may have to do with the pains—they *are not* themselves pains.

The pain-in-the-foot is thus *neither* in the physical space of the foot *nor* is it in the physical space of the brain, because pains are neither anatomical things like sinews, bones, or neurons, nor are they physiological processes such as charge-transfers on neuronal cell membranes. Where is the pain then? The answer is that it is in the "foot as a part of the living body," because this unified living body also produces—not least by means of the brain—*a spatially extended body subjectivity*. The fact that I can state meaningfully: "I have pains in my foot" and can also show the doctor the same foot presupposes that the subjective space of my pain and the objective space of my foot do not belong to two separate worlds but *coincide syntopically*.

This is certainly difficult to accept for a physicalist thinking. Is it not true that the "ghost in the machine" (Ryle 1949) is here being wakened again? Is it intended to allow the soul a secret readmission into the physically cleansed world? Indeed, it was a self-evident part of Aristotelian and pre-modern belief that the soul was indivisible and yet coextensive with the organic body.[8] Even Kant in his pre-critical period still wrote:

> I would, therefore, keep to common experience, and would say, provisionally, where I sense, there I am. I am just as immediately in the tips of my fingers, as in my head. It is myself who suffers in the heel and whose heart beats in affection. I feel the most painful impression when my corn torments me, not in a cerebral nerve, but at the end of my toes. No experience teaches me to believe some parts of my sensation to be removed from myself, to shut up my Ego into a microscopically small place in my brain from whence it may move the levers of my body-machine, and cause me to be thereby affected. Thus I should demand a strong proof to make inconsistent what the school-masters say: my soul is as a whole in my whole body, and wholly in each part. (Kant 1766/1900: 49)

If the phenomenal experience of lived body space is related to intersubjective and, hence, objective space, this is in fact linked to some extent to the doctrines of a co-extensivity of "soul" and "body," admittedly with quite a different terminology. Descartes argued against this, saying the body was only a machine of

---

[8] See Aristotle, De Anima 411 b 24: "In each of the bodily parts there are present all the parts of the soul." (http://classics.mit.edu/Aristotle/soul.html). Similar statements are found, for example, in Thomas Aquinas: "*Anima hominis est tota in toto corpore eius et iterum tota in qualibet parte ipsius*" (Thomas Aquinas 2009: I, q 93 a 3).

parts and thus divisible like a corpse, whereas the soul represents an indivisible whole.[9] It is not necessary, however, to reanimate Descartes's independent soul substance in order to reconcile the experience of our lived bodily being-in-the-world with an objective view of the physical body. The pre-condition is much rather an *adequate concept of life*: the organism itself represents a functional whole which is, as such, indivisible and, at the same time, extended in physical space—in parallel to the subjective body and its indivisible extension. An adequate concept of the living must therefore include the organismic-bodily as well as the subjective-bodily aspect. The two aspects are not simply externally connected with each other in the brain; rather, the living being as a whole appears, on the one hand, as a living, feeling, and expressive body[10] and, on the other, as a living organism.

The fact that this whole living organism can become the bearer of a likewise spatially ex-tended subjectivity does not add any new entity or soul substance to the physically describable world. No physical laws are thereby contradicted. However, it means a fundamental change for ourselves as living beings: we are no longer self-contained monads in the brain, for whom an image of the world is feigned, but rather *we inhabit our body and, by means of that, the world*. Phenomenology can thus put our primary experience in its rightful place again, namely to be in the world as incarnated beings.

Conclusion: Life-World and Neuroscience

The body is the center and the foundation of the life-world. Through its extensive spatiality, mobility, and dexterity we are embedded in the world and at home in it. Through its appearance, movements, and expression we also become perceptible and understandable as persons for others. It is what Husserl (1989) called the *personalistic* or life-worldly attitude in which we experience each other as embodied subjects. In the life-world, we do not meet each other as body vehicles in whose brains we locate the thoughts and feelings of the other, but as persons who inhabit their bodies, appear in them, and express themselves.

Already the dualism of Descartes, but also today's neurobiological constructivism rests on a twofold "disembodiment." On the one hand, the subjective body is objectivized as a mere physical thing; on the other hand, the bodily subject is

---

[9] Meditations VI (Descartes 2008: 60–1).

[10] In the perception of a pain-distorted face, the pain also becomes accessible from the perspective of the second person, thus again proving to be a phenomenon that does not belong to a virtual inner world but to the living and visible body as a whole.

hypostasized as a pure ego-consciousness and enclosed in a mental inner world. The body can then be explored from the observer's or third-person perspective; the conscious subject is left with only the undeniable but inaccessible first-person perspective. What is thus omitted is, on the one hand, the life-worldly or participant perspective, the *perspective of the second person*; on the other hand, the *principle of life*, which belongs to the organism as a whole. Neurobiological reductionism then results from a short circuit between the first- and third-person perspective, namely between the abstracted consciousness and the objectified body or brain as its *pars pro toto*. But it is not the brain that feels, thinks, perceives, or moves, but only the living being, the living organism as a whole.

As it turns out, corporeality is the key and at the same time the Achilles' heel of neurobiological reductionism. In order to cleanse the physical world of all experience and animation, the subjective body must be declared the internal construct of the brain; its spatial expansion must be only an illusion. In contrast to this, I have shown that subject- and object-body represent a "physical-aesthesiological unity," as Husserl (1989: 163) puts it, or in other words, that the subjectively experienced body and the intersubjectively perceived, physical body syntopically coincide. This body is of course no longer the divisible machine body of mechanistic physiology and medicine: the unity of the subjective body corresponds rather to the indivisible unity of the living organism. A refoundation of the concept of life on the basis of bodily self-awareness and of a systemic biology is therefore the central prerequisite for overcoming the naturalistic division of the person into physical and mental.[11]

The subject is extended over physical space, not in the form of a phantom image, a brain construct, but as subjectivity embedded in a living body and coextensive with it. The somatosensory and motor structures in the brain are, of course, necessary conditions for this subjective experience. But this does not mean that the body subject can be located in the brain like Descartes' soul in the pineal gland. We belong to the world, with skin and bone—we are physical, living, and therefore more "organic" beings than neuroscientific cerebrocentrism suggests. Neurobiology disregards the primacy of the life-worldly or participant perspective, from which alone the living and the lived body can be perceived. Instead, it ultimately advocates a metaphysical realism which believes it can recognize the "brain itself" and which regards life-worlds as mere constructs.

In contrast to the observer perspective, the participant perspective is the one from which people perceive each other as persons and communicate with

[11] On this, see my approach in "Ecology of the Brain" (Fuchs 2018).

each other. A person's experiencing, perceiving, feeling, and acting can only be grasped from this perspective; and only then, with certain restrictions, may it also be correlated with neuroscientific findings. He who does not know what "seeing" is and is unable to communicate with other sighted people about it, is also unable to explore the neurophysiology of optical perception. The very constitution of the object of neuroscientific research therefore requires the neuroscientist to adopt the participant perspective. "Without the intersubjectivity of understanding there can be no objectivity of knowledge" (Habermas 2004: 885).

In the second person perspective, we encounter each other as embodied subjects, as living beings with a body that is not a brain construct, either from an inner or outer perspective, but rather a physical-experiential unity. And just as there is no body in the brain, there are no brainworlds, no "cosmos in the head." Because the cosmos, as Heraclitus said, is not an *ídios kósmos*, a subjective inner world, but the *koinós kósmos*, the world we share with others. Reality is more than "the indifferent inner perspective of individuals who have the illusion of being subjects" (Spaemann 2011: 293; trans. T. F.). It is constituted in the mutual perception and recognition of individuals who know that they are not only the construct of the other and the other is not theirs. And as the other becomes real for us in his body, we also become real for ourselves, as bodily beings appearing in their bodies. Embodiment, life-world, and reality mutually ground each other.

References

Blanke, O., T. Metzinger. 2008. "Full-body illusions and minimal phenomenal selfhood." *Trends in Cognitive Sciences* **13**(1): 7–13.

Botvinick, M., J. Cohen. 1998. "Rubber hands 'feel' touch that eyes see." *Nature* **391** (6669): 756.

Crick, F. 1994. *The Astonishing Hypothesis: The Scientific Search for the Soul.* New York: Simon & Schuster.

Damasio, A. 1999. "How the brain creates the mind." *Scientific American* **281**: 112–117.

Descartes, R. 2008. *Meditations on First Philosophy.* **Michael Moriarty** (trans.) Oxford: Oxford University Press. (First published 1641.)

Descartes, R. 1989. *The Passions of the Soul.* **S. H. Voss** (trans.) Indianapolis/Cambridge: Hackett. (First published 1649.)

Eagleman, D. 2015. *Incognito: The Secret Lives of the Brain.* New York: Pantheon Books.

Fuchs, T. 2018. *Ecology of the Brain. The Phenomenology and Biology of the Embodied Mind.* Oxford: Oxford University Press.

Habermas, J. 2004. "Freiheit und Determinismus." *Deutsche Zeitschrift für Philosophie* **52**(6): 871–890.

Husserl, E. 1962. *Die Krisis der europäischen Wissenschaften und die transzendentale Phänomenologie*. Husserliana VI. Den Haag: Martinus Nijhoff.

Husserl, E. 1989. *Ideas Pertaining to a Pure Phenomenology and to a Phenomenological Philosophy II*. R. Rojcewicz, A. Schuwer (trans.) Dordrecht, Boston: Kluwer.

Kant, I. 1900. *Dreams of a Spirit-Seer*. [1766] London: Swan Sonnenschein & CO.

Katz, D. 1921. *Zur Psychologie des Amputierten und seiner Prothese*. E. F. Goerwitz (trans.) Leipzig: Barth.

Merleau-Ponty, M. 1962. *Phenomenology of Perception*. Colin Smith (trans.) London: Routledge & Kegan Paul.

Metzinger, T. 1999. *Subjekt und Selbstmodell*. 2. Aufl. Paderborn: Mentis.

Metzinger, T. 2009. *The Ego Tunnel: The Science of the Mind and the Myth of the Self*. New York: Basic Books.

Noë, A. 2009. *Out of Our Heads: Why You Are Not your Brain, and other Lessons from the Biology of Consciousness*. New York: Hill & Wang.

Ramachandran, V. S., S. Blakeslee. 1998. *Phantoms in the Brain: Probing the Mysteries of the Human Mind*. New York: William Morrow.

Ryle, G. 1949. *The Concept of Mind*. London: Hutchinson & Co.

Searle, J. R. 1992. *The Rediscovery of the Mind*. Cambridge/Mass.: MIT Press.

Seth, A. 2021. *Being You: A New Science of Consciousness*. New York: Dutton Books.

Spaemann, R. 2011. *Schritte über uns hinaus. Gesammelte Reden und Aufsätze II*. Stuttgart: Klett-Cotta.

Swaab, D. F. 2014. *We are our brains: A neurobiography of the brain, from the womb to Alzheimer's*. London: Penguin.

Thomas Aquinas 2009. *Summa theologica*. Latin-English edition, Vol. 2. Ypsilanti, Michigan: NovAntiqua.

Chapter 7

Perception and Reality: Sketch of an Interactive Realism

Introduction

Hardly any other age has so little confidence in perception as the present one. Already, in kindergarten, children are confronted with experiments, measurements, and sensory illusions as part of a science-oriented pedagogy that changes their intuitive access to the world into an experimental or constructivist approach. As early as possible, children are to transform themselves into "little researchers" who trust experiments more than their perceptions. For adults, as we have already seen in Chapter 6, neuroconstructivism provides the insight that perception only creates a more or less illusory world, namely a neuronal simulation of physical reality:

> The world around you, with its rich colors, textures, sounds, and scents is an illusion, a show put on for you by your brain [...] If you could perceive reality as it really is, you would be shocked by its colorless, odorless, tasteless silence. (Eagleman 2015: 38)

> Conscious experience is like a tunnel. [...] First, our brains generate a world-simulation, so perfect that we do not recognize it as an image in our minds. Then, they generate an inner image of ourselves as a whole [...] We are not in direct contact with outside reality or with ourselves [...] We live our conscious lives in the Ego Tunnel. (Metzinger 2009: 6–7)

According to this neuroconstructivist view, the real world is dramatically different from the one we experience. What we perceive are not the things themselves but only images or representations that they evoke in the brain. The real world is a rather desolate place of energy fields and particle movements, devoid of all qualities. The billionfold flickering of neuronal excitations creates my illusion of an outside world, while in truth I remain locked up in the cavity of my skull. This now widespread understanding of our experience as a "movie-in-the-brain" (Damasio 1999: 117) leads unsurprisingly to an epistemological (neuro-)solipsism. Because, how we communicate with others about our perceptions, when we ourselves perceive these others as mere brain-generated simulations, remains an unsolved question.

In Defense of the Human Being. Thomas Fuchs, Oxford University Press. © Suhrkamp Verlag 2021. DOI: 10.1093/oso/9780192898197.003.0008

Fortunately, our perception does not allow itself to be disconcerted by such "enlightenment"; for the time being, the common reality of the world is preserved. From a phenomenological point of view, Merleau-Ponty has emphasized what he calls "perceptual faith" (*foi perceptive*) as a kind of realism that is necessarily inherent in our perceptions:

> We see the things themselves, the world is what we see: formulae of this kind express a faith common to the natural man and the philosopher— the moment he opens his eyes; they refer to a deep-seated set of mute "opinions" implicated in our lives. (Merleau-Ponty 1968: 3)

This belief implies at the same time the intersubjective validity of perception: we always assume that others can also see what we see—we "take it for true," as the German term *Wahrnehmung* literally means. "And it is this unjustifiable certitude of a sensible world common to us that is the seat of truth within us" (ibid.: 11). Apparently, despite all attempts to refute it, the realism of perception cannot be abolished, as the phenomenological psychiatrist Erwin Straus has noted (not without irony): "It seems that naïve realism is reborn with each generation. The number of its followers exceeds the number of all other philosophical schools, and that without any effort of instruction and promotion" (Straus 1963: 952; trans. T. F.).

But is this commonality of the sensual world really "not to be justified," as Merleau-Ponty says? Are we left with only a doctrine of "double truth,"[1] the naive life-worldly and the scientifically enlightened truth? In the following, I will take a realistic (though not naively so) counter position to the conceptions of a world model simulated by the brain. I will argue that the experienced world is not an illusion, a model or a construct; we see, hear or feel the things themselves, not their representatives, images, or representations. Because perception, according to my first thesis, is neither an activity of the brain nor a process in a mental inner world, but rather an active engagement of living beings with their environment, or in short: *perception means sensorimotor interaction.*

But human perception is even more than that. Only humans are able to grasp objects and situations *as such*, i.e., independently of a purely subjective perspective. This is based on the ability—in evolutionary terms fundamentally unprecedented—to concur with the perspective of others: in a sense, we see, hear, feel, and handle things with the eyes, ears, and hands of others too. The objectivity or realism of perception results, according to the second thesis, from an *implicit intersubjectivity*. In early childhood, this inter-subjectivity arises

---

[1] This is the name given to the distinction between a "lower," philosophical and a "higher," theological truth, as advocated by certain scholastic philosophers of the Middle Ages.

above all in the formation of joint attention and joint action and is inscribed in perception—in short: *human perception results from interaction with others.*

This leads to the third thesis: for us, the fundamental reality is not the world of measurable quantities and particles abstracted by the special sciences, in particular physics, but the common reality of the life-world constituted by implicit intersubjectivity. The "taking for true" of human perception is based not only on the reliability of our sensorimotor contact with the environment but also on a collective frame of reference in which each individual perception is embedded. In place of a naïve realism or the supposedly mind-independent reality of physicalism, I thus argue for *a realism of the life-world.*

Perception as Interaction

According to the current cognitive science model, perception is an internal representation of the outside world in the brain, which thus creates the experience of the three-dimensional, colored world. Perception can therefore be analyzed as a linear-causal process that starts with an object as the cause and finally finds its goal in the representation of the object in the brain via the transmission of "sense data" and their neural processing. Thus, there is a preceding "objective reality," but of which we can only gain indirect knowledge. What we perceive is not reality itself but only its representatives in the inner world of consciousness—images, representations, models, or simulations. This theory of perception ultimately corresponds to the model of scientific knowledge: subject (inner world) and object (outer world) remain fundamentally separate from one another.

This representationalist view of perception ultimately goes back to the modern conception of consciousness, namely as an interior space or container in which the images of things are placed. Already with Descartes, every possible object of *res cogitans* or consciousness is an "idea"—a thought, a representation, or an image. Moreover, what we perceive are also images and not the things themselves. Subjective idealism is the philosophy which, in the wake of Descartes, develops from the image-theory of perception. For Locke, Hume and Kant, our perceptions are "impressions," "ideas," or "representations" from which we can only draw problematic conclusions about the reality in which we believe we are living. The idealist sits in the enclosure of his consciousness and receives the *ideae* as the delegates and representatives of things which he never gets to see themselves. In Locke's words:

> For, methinks, the understanding is not much unlike a closet wholly shut from light, with only some little openings left, to let in external visible resemblances, or ideas of things without. (Locke 1689/1997: 158)

To the present day, all internalistic, representationalist, or constructivist theories of perception have been derived from this idealistic conception. Searle has recently pointed out the fundamental fallacy to which they are all subject: here, the intentional object of perception—the seen *tree itself*—is confused with perception as a conscious process, i.e., with *my seeing the tree*, so that the tree now seems to become the mere content of my consciousness (cf. Searle 2015: 24–29). Under this assumption, one can be tempted by the misconception that we only see images of trees and not the trees themselves. Admittedly, my "seeing the tree" is different from the tree as such—if only because I see it from a certain perspective; but what I see is nevertheless the tree itself and not a "seen tree." In other words: there is no representative, no image of the tree "in my consciousness."

In contrast to such idealistic theories, interactive conceptions of perception were already developed in Jakob von Uexküll's and Viktor von Weizsäcker's theories of *functional* and *gestalt circles* (von Uexküll 1920/1973; von Uexküll 2001; von Weizsäcker 1940/1986). They are now reappearing in the concepts of *embodied and enactive cognition*, which we have already learned about (Varela et al. 1991; O'Regan & Noë 2001; Noë 2004; Thompson 2007). Here, perception is not a transformation of external stimuli into an inner model of the world, but rather an active, sensorimotor disclosure of the environment, motivated by the interests of the living being. In perception, a living being is not in opposition to the world, but entangled with it, as it were. *Perceivers are always participants in the world.* This requires first of all a mobile organism, as is already obvious from the word "perceive" (from Lat. *capere* = to seize): perception is only possible for a being that is able to move and grasp something, in other words, that has *agency*.

Hence, the activity of perception lies not only in attention. What a living being perceives also depends on its movement, and how it moves depends on its perceptions. According to the sensorimotor theory of O'Regan & Noë (2001) and Noë (2004), perception is the skillful dealing with objects in which the organism continuously relates the changes in sensory stimuli to its own movement: our gaze sweeps over the environment and thus provides the basis for our visual perception. The touching hand is guided by the shape and structure of the object, while conversely this structure is felt by the hand's movements. In addition, we always perceive objects as possibilities of grasping and handling, i.e., with their "invitation characters" (Lewin 1936) or "affordances" (Gibson 1979). An object such as forceps can only be perceived as such by an embodied being that is able to deal with it, for instance, one with suitable limbs to approach the forceps, to grasp it, and to grasp something with it.

In these functional cycles of perception and action, the sensory system already anticipates the motor function and, via movement, receives continuous feedback from the environment. Hence, receptivity and spontaneity as well as "inside" and "outside" can no longer be separated from each other. But this means that the basic prerequisite of representationalism of perception no longer applies. Because representations always stand "for something" from which they themselves must be separate or at least separable. If, however, the world is constituted for us only in constant interaction with it, if we are always already *acting* in the world, then there is no longer a separable "inside" that could reproduce, reconstruct, or re-present the "outside." In a continuous, interactive, circular process, no segment can stand for "another"—even if the circle runs through the brain. In this enactive conception, which I contrast to representationalism, acquired and flexible schemata of sensorimotor interaction with the environment take the place of representations.[2] Of course, cognition also includes the neuronal networks formed for this purpose but is only realized in circular processes that are fed back to the environment. In these interactions, the brain functions as a mediating or *relational organ* (Fuchs 2018), not as an internal producer of perception.

Accordingly, the *development* of the perceptive faculty is also based on interaction, i.e., on movement and action in the environment. This already applies to the perception of space. In a classical experiment, Held & Hain (1963) showed that newborn kittens, who are blind at first, cannot develop any spatial perception if during the first weeks of life they are only carried around and not allowed to move themselves. Although they were exposed to the same visual stimuli as other kittens, they did not learn to see spatially without movement. This means that only the sentient and *at the same time moving* organism forms the experiential space, namely from the coherently linked patterns of motor and sensory functions including the sense of balance.

Even something as basic as space can only be experienced by embodied and acting beings. The enactive approach generalizes this insight: the experienced world emerges for us in the course of our interaction with it. Perception has objectivity because it is formed *in the world for the world*, both phylogenetically and ontogenetically. In ontogenesis, this interaction includes the formation of the brain structures required to adequately perceive the environment. This has been impressively demonstrated in experiments by the neuroscientist Mriganka Sur and his research team (Melchner et al. 2000). They severed the

---

[2] Representations can only be spoken of in the case of secondary ideas, fantasies or memories that are evoked independently of perception.

optic nerve of newborn ferrets (which are born blind) so that the stump grew together with the part of the diencephalon that otherwise transmits impulses from the *auditory* nerve to the auditory center in the cortex. Now visual stimuli reached a brain region that normally processes acoustic signals. Surprisingly, however, with the ferrets moving in their environment, the brain area gradually adapted to the new sensory input: stimulated by regularly linked visual and motor afferences, the auditory center turned into a visual center. Even nerve cells characteristic of a visual center were formed, so that after a few weeks the ferrets were able to see with the respective eye.

From these insights we can derive the following principle: it is not the brain that generates the function, but conversely *the function, in its embodied execution, that creates its cerebral organ*. Hence, the astonishing healing powers of the brain: even after serious brain lesions, the functions of speech, memory, and orientation can be taken over by the other hemisphere, namely *by the patient practicing these functions* (Maier et al. 2019). Through sensory, motor, as well as mental activity, network structures are formed in the brain that are suitable for the function. They are then closed into a complete functional circuit each time the organism encounters and interacts with a corresponding situation in the environment.

The Objectifying Power of Perception

Perception and movement are thus linked to each other in continuous circular processes, and in perception the living being forms a comprehensive system with its environment. In other words: the carrier processes, which are necessary for perceptual experiences, continually cross the boundaries of the brain and the body. We have thus substantiated the first thesis mentioned at the beginning: *perception means sensorimotor interaction with the environment.*

This interactive concept replaces the notion of internal representations, yet one might still ask: if perception is based on interaction, even on an entanglement of living beings and environment, how does the "opposition" come about in which things present themselves to us in perception? After all, as Hans Jonas rightly states, in every perception "[...] external objects are apprehended not merely as 'such', but also as 'there'. [...] Perception is intrinsically awareness of such a self-giving presence – the experience of the reality of the object as co-existing with me here and now" (Jonas 1966: 168).

The answer to this question lies in a principle that Hegel described in his logic as "mediated immediacy" (Hegel 1812/1979: 115): in perception, the mediating sensorimotor processes allow what is perceived "to shine through," as it were; these processes become *transparent*. Although perceptual consciousness is formed on the basis of the entire process of interaction, it is only directed at the object itself, which thus appears to us in its immediacy—as real. In this sense, the body with its sensations and movements can also be understood as the medium *through which* we perceive the world, but which itself fades into the background.

Already on the *physiological* level, various mechanisms contribute to this self-concealment of the body in perception: for example, the motor activity of the eye is taken into account and balanced by so-called *efference copies* in the sensory system.[3] Otherwise, with every eye movement, the environment seen would also begin to fluctuate (if, on the other hand, one closes one eye and now moves the other eyeball with a slight lateral finger pressure from the outside—a physiologically "unintended" eye movement—then one actually sees the environment fluctuating back and forth!).[4] Similarly, in phenomenal experience, the mediality of the body shows itself in the fact that we usually transcend the mediating or "proximal" sensations to the "distal" objects and situations.[5] It is in this sense that Heidegger writes:

> Much closer to us than all sensations are the things themselves. We hear the door slamming in the house and never hear acoustic sensations or even mere noises. To hear a pure sound, we have to listen away from things, pull our ear away from them, i.e. hear abstractly. (Heidegger 1935/1977: 10 f.; trans. T. F.)

Likewise, we are usually not consciously aware of our eye movements, we are already *with* the things we fix our eyes upon. The same principle applies to touching: every tactile sensation is first and foremost an affection of the body

---

[3] In this process, a draft of movement in the brain is passed on "in copy" to sensory areas even before the motor activity is triggered, so that these areas "subtract" the movement from the sensory feedback from the environment that arrives later; see Holst and Mittelstaedt (1950).

[4] This is just one example of the many physiological mechanisms by which perception conveys a coherent reality. The sensory illusions repeatedly cited since antiquity to justify skepticism are also based on the fact that perception does not merely provide "1:1 impressions" or "photographic images" of physical stimuli, but rather enables us to orient ourselves in the environment, to recognize real things, and to deal with them. Perception therefore produces, for example, constants of form or color even where the field of perception is discontinuous or distorted (for example, we do not see an inclined rectangle as a rhombus, but always as a rectangle; a red rose remains red even at dusk, etc.). It emphasizes contrasts, distinguishes foreground and background, completes ambiguous contours to form *gestalten*, and compensates for perspective distortions. The resulting so-called illusions are thus based on highly meaningful adaptations of perception to the requirements of a living being of medium size who is mobile and who orientates itself in the world.

[5] For the terms "proximal" and "distal" in this context, see Polanyi (1966).

at its interfaces. But it is precisely this affection that enables us to feel an object, i.e., to grasp its surface structure, extension, position, and so on. Trained blind persons are even able to read a text by touching the dots of Braille, i.e., to direct themselves *through their fingers* toward intentional content—just as sighted people do by glancing at a page.

Thus, through the affections of their body, perceiving subjects are directed toward the reality of the things that appear to them, or in other words, they perceive bodily sensory complexes *as* the objects of their world.[6] The same applies to the *acting* subject: by means of the body—often the hand—we pursue our goals of action, usually without becoming aware of our body at all. Indeed, in skillful handling of objects, for example playing the piano or driving a car, we incorporate these instruments so that they in turn become the media of our actions. This is why an experienced driver can feel the grip or slipperiness of the road under the wheels of his car, just as a blind person feels the ground at the tip of his stick and not in his hand.

This now indicates a form of *implicit linkage* in perception, "... in which the mediating link is necessary in order to establish the immediacy of the connection" (Plessner 1928/1975: 324; trans. T. F.). Perception and action mean our "being toward the world" (Merleau-Ponty) through the tacitly mediating, implicit medium of the body. In our perceptions we are always already beyond the body; we grasp in mediated immediacy what presents itself through the body as the content of experience. This content is neither sensory data nor signs, neither pictures nor representations, but rather a relational reality that is grasped relative to us and yet is directly experienced.

The Implicit Intersubjectivity of Perception

Perception thus means the mediated immediacy of our relationship to the world. However, it is also true that we humans, unlike animals, know about the indirectness of our relationship to the world: whatever we perceive or do, we can always reflect on the perception of what is perceived, or on the execution of the action itself, withdraw our attention from distal goals, as it were, and direct

---

[6] Cf. once again Jonas: "But there is this paradox to sense perception: the felt affectiveness of its data, which is necessary for the experience of the 'reality' of the real, [...] must in part be canceled out again in order to permit the apprehension of its 'objectivity'. The element of encounter is balanced by one of abstraction, without which sensation would not rise to perception. [...] there is 'abstraction' from the state of sensory stimulation itself in the very fact of perceiving the object instead of one's own organic affection. [...] In that appearance the affective basis ('stimulation', 'irritation') is canceled, its record neutralized" (Jonas 1966: 168).

it toward proximal mediations. According to Plessner, this can ultimately lead to a situation where:

> [...] man begins to doubt the immediacy of his knowledge, the directness of his real contact, as it exists for him with absolute evidence. [...] Of course, then it is said, the subject means to grasp reality and to have it himself. But that is only true for the subject. Factually, it moves among the contents of consciousness, ideas and sensations. (Plessner 1928/1975: 329; trans. T. F.)

Nietzsche had already formulated this in his influential critique of knowledge:

> Around every being there is a concentric circle with a center, which is peculiar to it. Similarly, the ear encloses us in a small space, similarly the sense of touch. According to these horizons, in which, as in prison walls, our senses enclose each of us, we now measure the world, we call this near and that far, this large and that small, this hard and that soft [...] We are in our web, we spiders, and whatever we catch in it, we cannot catch anything but what can be caught in *our* web! (Nietzsche 1899: 1092 f.; trans. T. F.)

The neuroconstructivist theory of knowledge outlined at the beginning is also based on this skepticism: the world then appears only as an internal construct of the perceptual system or the brain. But, with this notion, the baby is thrown out with the bath water. For it is precisely the relativization of the purely subjective impression, which we as humans can make by means of reflection, that makes the actual *objectivity* of our perception possible. The ability to reflect means, at the same time, the possibility to implicitly take into account the point of view of others or of the "generalized other" (Mead 1934).

Let us look at this more closely. Perception gives us things in perspective yet as they are, as objects, independent of our mere sight or momentary impression. Berkeley's "*esse est percipi*" certainly does not correspond to our perceptual experience—no one would think that things only appeared with their perception and that without them they would disappear into nothingness. How is that possible? Here I come now to the second thesis put forward at the beginning: the objectifying performance of human perception is due to an *implicit intersubjectivity*. The things that I perceive are at the same time always fundamentally perceptible and attainable for others as well, i.e., in principle available for joint action. Through the implicit participant perspective (the "we" perspective), my subjective perception acquires its fundamental objectivity (even if it must be corrected in individual cases). In other words: human perception is intersubjectively constituted. I will explain this in more detail in the following.

What we perceive are neither pictures nor models, but things and people. At first this is by no means self-evident: when I perceive a table, for example, I only ever see it from one, particularly limited, perspective. Husserl has shown, however, that perception overcomes its own perspective to the extent that it integrates current and other possible perspectives. The different views ("adumbrations") of a table, the various sides, the hidden back, but also the table's materiality are implicitly seen or "appresented," as Husserl puts it, so that I see *the table itself* and not a mere impression or a subjective image (Husserl 1966: 3–24; 1984: 588 f.).

But these implicitly witnessed views also contain a latent intersubjectivity: the table that I see there is an object that, at the same time, *others could see from other angles*. Thus, the object gains its actual objectivity only through the possibility of being perceived by different subjects—in other words, through an implicitly presupposed diversity of other perspectives. Husserl also speaks here of the "horizon of possible own and foreign experience" or of an "open intersubjectivity" (Husserl 1973: 289; cf. Zahavi 2001: 53ff.). In a similar way, according to Sartre—who refers back to Husserl here—an object is not constituted for a pure subject, but always in a context of reference in which the others are included:

> Whether I consider this table or this tree or this bare wall in solitude or with companions, the Other is always there as a layer of constitutive meanings which belong to the very object which I consider; in short, he is the veritable guarantee of the object's objectivity. […] Thus each object, far from being constituted as for Kant, by a simple relation to the subject, appears in my concrete experience as polyvalent; it is given originally as possessing systems of reference to an indefinite plurality of consciousnesses; it is on the table, on the wall that the Other is revealed to me as that to which the object under consideration is perpetually referred – as well as on the occasion of the concrete appearances of Pierre or Paul. (Sartre 1956: 233)

However, as Merleau-Ponty emphasizes, the perceiving subject always experiences not only the object but also *himself* as perceptible to others:

> As soon as I see, it is necessary that the vision […] be doubled with a complementary vision or with another vision; myself seen from without, such as another would see me, installed in the midst of the visible, occupied in considering it from a certain spot. (Merleau-Ponty 1968: 134)

Human perception, as these reflections can be summarized, is not a lonely relationship of a subject to the world. It always contains the possible presence and the possible perspectives of others—even Robinson Crusoe saw his island with the eyes of others, even before Friday came along. The objects of perception not only exist "for me," but have always been collectively constituted. This ability to share one's own perceptions with others in principle, however, simultaneously enables the subject to distance himself from the object of perception—it allows for an *objectification*. Plessner already came to the same conclusion: the specific sociality of humans, namely the self's ability to adopt the others' perspective, is the reason for our "eccentric position" in the world and with it, for "the distance demanded by reality, so that it can manifest itself [. . .], the scope in which alone reality can appear" (Plessner 1928/1975: 331; trans. T. F.).

(Neuro-)constructivism thus fails to recognize the objectivization that human perception achieves as implicit intersubjective perception, because it only considers the individual processes of stimulus transmission from the object to the respective brain. Since each brain, according to neuroconstructivist assumptions, only creates its own virtual space, there can be no "common simulation space" or "ego tunnel" between two individuals. This would have the consequence, as we have already seen in Chapter 6, that two people could not jointly view one and the same object.

But, in every interaction and understanding with others we refer to a common space, to jointly intended objects, and situations. For instance, each everyday act of exchange in the marketplace presupposes that we are not dealing with inner images in our interaction. The banknote I hold in my hand is not my subjective imagination but rather the note seen and received by the seller. Buyer and seller thus participate in the intersubjective and thereby objective space of common objects. The processes of mediation on which their perception is based become transparent for a jointly intended reality that transcends subjectivism. In seeing or perceiving, we have always already found ourselves in a common world. In place of a "naive realism" we can therefore set forth a *life-worldly realism*.

Genesis of Intersubjective Perception

Even if Husserl takes for granted a transcendental intersubjectivity of perception, empirically speaking, the *genesis* of this structure can hardly be doubted: it is what each of us learns and acquires in the course of early childhood through social interactions. Human perception is neither given a priori nor is it a merely natural process; it is instead a perception that is socialized or *cultivated* in situations of shared attention and practice, i.e., in situations of jointly directed action or "we-intentionality." Just as the sensorimotor space is formed through interaction with the *physical* environment (as we saw in the experiment with the newborn kittens), so the objective or intersubjective space of human perception is constituted in the course of *social* interaction.[7]

Perceiving things as such presupposes stepping out of the primary, subject-centered reference to a situation, and thus a mobility of perspective, which is learned in typical, *triadic* social interactions (Fuchs 2013). From the eighth to

---

[7] Cf. Vygotsky (1978: 57): "Every function in the child's cultural development appears twice: first, on the social level, and later, on the individual level; first, *between* people (*interpsychological*), and then *inside* the child (*intrapsychological*)."

the ninth month of life onwards, babies begin to turn to objects together with adults (joint attention, see Tomasello 1999: 56 ff.). They learn to understand each other's pointing gestures, they themselves start pointing at things and make sure that the adults are paying attention by short glances. Pointing involves a common reference to a third entity—hence "triadic"—which is seen or handled by both partners, and both are aware of this common directionality.

Joint attention fundamentally transforms the attitude toward things as well as toward others. "Seen with others' eyes," things become *objects* in the etymological sense of the word, which are now given independently and at a distance from the primary subjective perspective. In Heidegger's terminology: things ready-to-hand (*zuhanden*) become objects present-at-hand (*vorhanden*). In order to show the object to an adult on the other hand, the child must grasp what this adult sees, i.e., at least implicitly follow his or her spatial perspective— a perspective that is no longer only dyadically directed at the child but also at the common environment, and which differs from its own. Object triangulation thus enables a shared or "we-intentionality" (Tomasello & Rakoczy 2003: 121), which gradually shapes the child's perception.

It is further supported by the *interactive handling* of objects: embedded in action contexts, the common reference to the object is validated by mutual interactions. The ball that the child sees is the ball that the child receives from and returns to the mother, with which they play together, and which is embedded in their intersubjective familiarity with the world. Perception is thus from the very beginning interactive and at the same time culturally shaped: plates, spoons, chairs, toys, clothes, shoes—almost everything that the child becomes familiar with are culturally shaped objects and correspondingly preformed performances.

An innate tendency of infants to learn from adults also contributes to the sociality of perception, which in current infant research is referred to as "natural pedagogy" (Csibra & Gergely 2009). So-called "ostensive cues" (eye contact, gestures, vocalizations) signal a learning context ("watch out, this is important!") to the child so that he or she understands the subsequent object-related action of the adult as significant and often tries to imitate it. In this way other people act as a source of attitudes toward things and events in the shared environment. There is also a phenomenon that developmental psychology calls "social referencing": if children of about 9 months of age are confronted with an object that is unknown to them and that causes uncertainty or fear, for instance a robot that moves toward them with a beeping sound, they will first look at the parents to determine whether they react anxiously or joyfully to the object, and then orientate their reaction toward the parents' reaction (Hornik et al. 1987;

Hirshberg & Svejda 1990). Each step of opening up the cultural world is thus based on a store of shared experience; things get their meaning for the child from the way they are handled by others. In this way the common life-world is constituted.

Joint attention and the associated pointing gesture is ultimately also the prerequisite for the acquisition of *language*. The first words are connected with the pointing gesture: the parents point to objects and name them; the children recognize that the parents use words with an intention to designate and begin to adopt them. This learning process is always embedded in cooperative activities: changing nappies, eating together, building a tower of blocks, and so on are the typical contexts in which the corresponding words are learned. The ability to speak thus develops in intersubjective actions, in practices directed toward the shared environment (Bruner 1983; Nelson 1996; Tomasello 2019: 112ff.).

With the acquisition of linguistic meanings, the child also acquires the implicit intersubjectivity of the "generalized other," which is also reflected in perception. By naming things, they enter the common sphere or inventory of symbolic meanings, which lends perception an expanded generality and objectivity. Because each perceived object now refers not only spatially to the possible perspectives of the others but also to a layer of jointly constituted and habitualized meanings, which are not added to the perceptions secondarily but are inscribed in them.

The linguistic-conceptual division and classification of the world is thus communicated to perception, namely as a *typification* ("lion," "tiger," "leopard") which we already see before we make an explicit designation such as "this is a tiger." What a tiger is, we have grasped in situations of joint attention and naming, and its concept has subsequently entered our perception as a scheme and type. So, we do not see any colors and forms that we then interpret as a tiger, but the sense-unit "tiger" is already perceptually given to us. This sense of the perceived is always related to the reference context of all things and their embedding in the common life-world, which in turn—now on the higher level of symbolically conveyed meanings—gives every perception its objective, i.e., intersubjectively valid reality.

Subjectivation of Perception in Schizophrenia

A look at pathological forms of experience in schizophrenia shows that the objectifying power of perception is not given once and for all—it can be lost again. Here, especially at the beginning of acute psychoses, there often occurs a radical and disturbing *subjectivation* of perception so that the patients only see *pictures of things* instead of the things themselves (Fuchs 2005). As a result, the environment appears unreal and artificial, as if it were staged just for them. At the same time, the familiar, intersubjectively constituted meanings of things and situations decompose:

> Everywhere you look, everything looks so unreal. The whole environment, everything becomes strange, and you get terribly scared. [...] Somehow everything is suddenly there for me, arranged for me. Everything around you suddenly refers to you. You're in the center of a plot, just like in the movies. (Klosterkötter 1988: 69)

> On the street, everything seemed strange and somehow eerie – as if a war had broken out or the world was coming to an end. [...] All the time cars were passing by as if they were fleeing from something; everything frightened me. The car signs were signals for something I had yet to decipher. I was looking for some kind of code. (Patient from my own clinic)

Such pathological forms of experience illustrate *ex negativo* the objectifying achievement of normal perception. Objectivity is not only conferred on perception by a subsequent judgement of its reality but is inherent in it as a "perceptual faith": perception transcends itself toward its object. In schizophrenia, on the other hand, patients no longer grasp the distal content "through their perception"; instead, the proximal, "subjective" process of perception itself enters into consciousness. In this way, the patients become, as it were, spectators of their own seeing:

> I *become aware* of my eye watching an object. (Stanghellini 2004: 113)

> I saw everything I did like a film camera. (Sass 1992: 132)

> For me it was as if my eyes were cameras, [...] but somehow as if my head were enormous, the size of the universe, and I was in the far back and the cameras were at the very front. (de Haan & Fuchs 2010: 329 f.)

Here, the subject is, as it were, placed outside the world; it literally becomes a homunculus in the head, regarding its own perceptions like projected images. It is *only in psychosis*, then, that the enclosure of consciousness, Locke's "closet," is created, in which the subject perceives merely the *ideae*, the images, and representations of things. This subjectivation can even reach the point where the patient believes that the existence of the perceived itself depends on his or her own perception—a pathological form of Berkeley's "*esse est percipi*":

> Whenever I took my eyes of them [the hospital guards], they disappeared. In fact, everything at which I did not direct my entire attention seemed not to exist. (Landis, 1964: 90; quoted in Sass 1992: 277 f.)

> If I perceive a door and then look away, then it's almost as if the door ceases to exist. (Henriksen 2011: 24)

In schizophrenia, as we can see, the perceptual being-in-the-world, the implicit intersubjectivity and thus objectivity of perception can be lost. The patients then involuntarily become "subjective idealists," even solipsists, who remain locked into their deficient perceptions like in a world of their own. But what we can recognize here is once again the objectification that normal perception provides. The "ego tunnel" in which we live according to the neuroconstructivist conception, the movie-in-the-head that is supposedly presented to us by our brain, is in reality only a pathological state that patients experience in psychosis (Fuchs 2020). In ordinary experience, on the other hand, we find ourselves in the shared world, constituted by the implicit intersubjectivity of perception.

The patient in the last case study also experienced an alienation of perception, namely a loss of "perceptual faith," which ultimately led to delusions of persecution:

> It seemed more and more unreal to me, like a foreign country. Then I got the idea that this isn't my old environment anymore. It couldn't be our house anymore. Someone could have set the stage for me. A backdrop, or someone has recorded a TV play for me. Then I scanned the walls. […] I checked to see if this was a real surface. (Klosterkötter 1988: 64 f.)

The subjectivation, and at the same time alienation of perception leaves this patient with nothing more than stage scenery, while we see things themselves in their constancy and reliability. This fundamental shake-up of perceptual faith, this "ontological doubt" can, from a certain point on, only be compensated for by delusion: the patient developed the conviction that a secret service was abusing her for experimental purposes and projecting fake images into her brain via radiation. The delusion thus represents a source of coherence and meaning in a mysteriously alienated world. But, at the same time, it means the loss of the implicit intersubjectivity of perception, the withdrawal from our common reality into a solipsistic world of one's own.[8]

Summary

The currently dominant naturalistic and constructivist theories of perception understand it as an internal representation or simulation of the outside world,

---

[8] Another potential way to demonstrate the objectifying power of perception would be an analysis of *dream consciousness*: here, too, there is a subjectivation and a loss of objectivity. The dreamer is passively placed in situations where he is center-stage, situations which consistently show an intense self-referential significance, even if this significance often remains mysterious. The dreamer is not in a position to transcend these situations towards a general perspective and thus to relativize them. In addition, he typically see only images, not objects.

which is generated in the brain from incoming sensory data. They thus ascribe a fundamentally illusory character to perception in relation to physical reality ("online simulation," "movie-in-the-head," "ego tunnel"). In contrast to this, I have formulated two theses which defend our primary "perceptual faith" and are capable of establishing a realism of perception in the real world, namely (1) an *enactivist*, and (2) a *social interactionist thesis*:

(1) Perception is based neither on a mere data transfer from the outside to the inside nor on internal modelling, but on a *continuous sensorimotor inter-action of living beings with their surroundings*. Every perception means an overarching coupling of organism and environment. Thus, the separation of inside and outside, which representationalism presupposes, is no longer tenable. The objectifying performance of perception results in this context from *mediated immediacy*, namely from the transparency of the mediating bodily processes for the distal contents of perception.

(2) Human perception overcomes its own perspectivity or self-centrality through an *implicit intersubjectivity*, i.e., by taking into account the possible perspectives of others. It is thus able to grasp objects and situations *as such*, i.e., in their independence from the act of perception. This implicit inter-subjectivity is based ontogenetically on early social interactions: joint at-tention, shared practice, and finally common language constitute a shared or "we-intentionality" that inscribes itself into individual perception and thus establishes its *life-worldly realism*.

On the first level of perception, which we have in common with animals, there is no concept of reality in the sense of distinguishing it from "unreality"—animals only experience real sensorimotor contact with the environment, which may fail but does not yet create a concept of "unreality" or appearance. Reality in the genuine sense only exists for humans. It is only from intersubjectivity that a universality results, which turns our perceptions and experiences into possible experiences of others. The perceived world is thereby constituted as an impli-citly intersubjective reality, which is thus legitimately entitled to the predicate of objectivity—an objectivity of perception that can always be corrected by fur-ther communication and comparison of perspectives with others, and which thus stands out from mere appearance.[9]

In conclusion, the third thesis put forward at the beginning of this chapter still needs to be substantiated: the life-worldly realism of perception can never be com-pletely replaced by the assumptions of scientific models or reduced to physical

---

[9] On the intersubjective alignment of perspectives as a prerequisite for the development of objectivity, compare also the summary account in Tomasello (2019), especially pp. 82–90.

processes. Because models only serve to ensure the proven calculability and pre-dictability of observable natural processes, and however successfully they fulfil these purposes, they cannot *qua models* describe an "actual" transphenomenal reality. Models are at bottom always of a hypothetical nature, they are valid as long as their predictions prove correct, and good models do so successfully. However, this does not mean that they are more "real" than the reality they are supposed to explain or predict. Rather, the validity of every observation of nature and every empirical research finding is itself based on the reality of the life-world, beyond which there can be no position of observation and knowledge. Habermas, for ex-ample, emphasized this in his critique of neuro-determinism:

> The objectivity of the world can only be constituted for an observer in conjunction with the intersubjectivity of a possible understanding of that which the observer cog-nitively grasps from inner-worldly events. Only the intersubjective verification of sub-jective evidence enables the progressive objectification of nature. For this reason, the processes of understanding cannot themselves be placed entirely on the object side, i.e. they cannot be described completely as inner-worldly determined events and thus be "captured" in an objectifying way. (Habermas 2004: 883; trans. T. F.)

The objectivity of knowledge thus rests on the intersubjectivity of symbolic pro-cesses of understanding. However, as we have seen, our directly experienced reality already implies the intersubjectivity of perception and, at the same time, draws its validation from it. Therein lies the life-worldly prerequisite for all sci-entific practice and knowledge.

Reductionist naturalism or physicalism is inconsistent in so far as it over-looks its own dependence on the intersubjectively constituted life-world. The life-world has a triadic relationship structure "I - You - It": as members of a communicative community, we are directed toward the objects of our envir-onment in joint attention. The scientific observer perspective, the perspective of the third person, is thus preceded by the participant or "we" perspective, to which scientific knowledge, as a special form of social practice, always remains bound. No physical object can be identified independently of intersubjective experience. What a brain, neurons, molecules, atoms, or energy fields are re-sults only from a common pre-understanding, from conventions, and scientific practice. It follows, however, that a *purely physically* conceived nature must re-main a theoretical construct from which consciousness, perception, and inter-subjectivity cannot be derived without remainder.

Dirk Hartmann has drawn attention to this "second naturalistic fallacy"[10] in reductionism. It consists in the fact that the material structures and processes

---

[10] The "second," since a naturalistic fallacy usually refers to the derivation of claims about what ought to be from statements about what is (Hume's "is-ought problem," or G. E. Moore's naturalistic fallacy).

postulated at the level of the scientific model or construct are now foisted onto experience in the life-world and then ultimately hypostasized into actual reality:

> A knife consists of a blade and a handle, the material of the blade is an alloy, it consists of molecules, which are a combination of atoms, which consist of even smaller particles – all just a matter of "taking a closer look." What is overlooked is that, unlike the objects of the phenomenal plane, the constructs are not accessible independently of the theories in which they occur. (Hartmann 1998: 326)

Constructs or models are not our perceptions, as neuroconstructivism claims, but rather the worlds of measurably describable particles, waves, and energy fields that have been abstracted from the special sciences, in particular, physics. In principle, these elude common perception and can only ever be plausibilized or falsified indirectly. Such constructs or models may well be successfully applied to the description and prediction of physical and physiological processes and thus undoubtedly capture aspects of the transphenomenal world. However, these aspects are only ever accessible to us in an indirect way, on the basis of shared perceptual experiences.

Thus, the same applies to intersubjective, life-worldly perception as Habermas showed applies to intersubjective processes of understanding: it cannot be placed completely on the object side. Physiological investigations can clarify the physical and organismic *conditions* of specific perceptions; but they cannot provide a sufficient *explanation* of perception as an interactive relationship between humans and their environment. For us, the fundamental reality is not the world of mathematically describable quantities, particles, or neuronal activities abstracted in the special sciences; it is rather the reality of the life-world constituted by implicit intersubjectivity. It would therefore make no sense to regard physical models, electrons, or quarks as more "real" than this jointly perceived reality. Instead, the validity of every empirical research finding rests itself on the reality of the life-world, beyond which there can be no position of observation and knowledge.

References

Bruner, J. 1983. *Child's Talk: Learning to Use Language.* Oxford: Oxford University Press.

Csibra, G., G. Gergely. 2009. "Natural pedagogy." *Trends in Cognitive Sciences* 13(4): 148–153.

Damasio, A. 1999. *The Feeling of what Happens. Body and Emotion in the Making of Consciousness.* New York: Hartcourt Brace & Co.

De Haan, S., T. Fuchs. 2010. "The ghost in the machine: Disembodiment in schizophrenia. Two case studies." *Psychopathology* 43(5): 327–333.

Eagleman, D. 2015. *Incognito: The Secret Lives of the Brain.* New York: Pantheon Books.

Fuchs, T. 2005. "Delusional mood and delusional perception. A phenomenological analysis." *Psychopathology* 38(3): 133–139.

Fuchs, T. 2013. "The phenomenology and development of social perspectives." *Phenomenology and the Cognitive Sciences* 12(4): 655–683.

Fuchs, T. 2018. *Ecology of the Brain. The phenomenology and Biology of the Embodied Mind.* Oxford: Oxford University Press.

Fuchs, T. 2020. "Delusion, reality and intersubjectivity: A phenomenological and enactive analysis." *Philosophy, Psychiatry & Psychology* 27: 61–79.

Gibson, J. 1979. *The Ecological Approach to Visual Perception.* Boston: Houghton Mifflin.

Habermas, J. 2004. "Freiheit und Determinismus." *Deutsche Zeitschrift für Philosophie* 52(6): 871–890.

Hartmann, D. 1998. *Philosophische Grundlagen der Psychologie.* Darmstadt: Wissenschaftliche Buchgesellschaft.

Hegel, G. F. W. 1979. Wissenschaft der Logik I. Erster Teil. Die objektive Logik. Erstes Buch. *Werke* Bd. 5. Frankfurt/M.: Suhrkamp. (Erstausgabe 1812.)

Heidegger, M. 1977. "Der Ursprung des Kunstwerkes." In *Holzwege.* Gesamtausgabe Bd. 5. F.-W. von Herrmann (ed.) Frankfurt/M.: Klostermann (pp. 1–74). (1st edition 1935.)

Held, R., A. Hein. 1963. "Movement-produced stimulation in the development of visually guided behavior." *Journal of Comparative Physiology and Psychology* 56(5): 872–876.

Henriksen, M. G. 2011. *Understanding Schizophrenia. Investigations in Phenomenological Psychopathology* (Dissertation). Copenhagen: Faculty of Health Sciences of Copenhagen University.

Hirshberg, L. M., M. Svejda. 1990 "When infants look to their parents: In infants' social referencing of mothers compared to fathers." *Child Development* 61(4): 1175–1186.

Holst, E. v., H. Mittelstaedt. 1950. "Das Reafferenzprinzip." *Naturwissenschaften* 37(20): 464–476.

Hornik, R., N. Risenhoover, M. Gunnar. 1987. "The effects of maternal positive, neutral, and negative affective communications on infant responses to new toys." *Child Development* 58(4): 937–944.

Husserl, E. 1966. *Analysen zur passiven Synthesis.* M. Fleischer (ed.). Husserliana XI. Den Haag: Martinus Nijhoff.

Husserl, E. 1973. *Zur Phänomenologie der Intersubjektivität. Texte aus dem Nachlass II. 1921-28.* I. Kern (ed.). Husserliana XIV. Den Haag: Martinus Nijhoff.

Husserl, E. 1984. *Logische Untersuchungen. II/2. Untersuchungen zur Phänomenologie und Theorie der Erkenntnis.* U. Panzer (ed.). Husserliana XIX/2. Den Haag: Martinus Nijhoff.

Jonas, H. 1966. *The Phenomenon of Life: Toward a Philosophical Biology.* New York: Harper & Row.

Klosterkötter, J. 1988. *Basissymptome und Endphänomene der Schizophrenie.* Berlin, Heidelberg, New York: Springer.

Landis, C. 1964. *Varieties of Psychopathological Experience.* New York: Holt, Rinehart & Winston.

Lewin, K. 1936. *Principles of Topological Psychology.* New York: McGraw-Hill.

Locke, J. 1997. *An Essay Concerning Human Understanding.* London: Penguin. (Originally published 1689.)

Maier, M., B. R. Ballester, P. F. Verschure. 2019. Principles of neurorehabilitation after stroke based on motor learning and brain plasticity mechanisms. *Frontiers in Systems Neuroscience* **13**: 74.

Mead, G. H. 1934. *Mind, Self and Society from the Standpoint of a Social Behaviorist.* Chicago: University of Chicago Press.

Melchner, L. V., S. L. Pallas, M. Sur. 2000. "Visual behavior mediated by retinal projections directed to the auditory pathway." *Nature* **404**(6780): 871–876.

Merleau-Ponty, M. 1968. *The Visible and the Invisible, followed by working notes.* Alphonso Lingis (trans.) Evanston: Northwestern University Press.

Metzinger, T. 2009. *The Ego Tunnel: The Science of the Mind and the Myth of the Self.* New York: Basic Books.

Nelson, K. 1996. *Language in Cognitive Development.* Cambridge: Cambridge University Press.

Nietzsche, F. W. 1899. *Morgenröthe. Gedanken über die moralischen Vorurtheile.* Nietzsche's Werke, Erste Abteilung, Bd. 4. Leipzig: E. G. Naumann.

Noë, A. 2004. *Action in Perception.* Cambridge, MA: MIT Press.

O'Regan, J. K., A. Noë. 2001. "A sensorimotor account of vision and visual consciousness." *Behavioral and Brain Sciences* **24**(5): 939–1011.

Plessner, H. 1975. *Die Stufen des Organizchen und der Mensch.* Berlin: De Gruyter. (1st edition 1928.)

Polanyi, M. 1966. *The Tacit Dimension.* Chicago: University of Chicago Press.

Sartre, J.-P. 1956. H. E. Barnes (trans.) *Being and Nothingness* (1943). New York: Philosophical Library.

Sass, L. A. 1992. *Madness and Modernism. Insanity in the Light of Modern Art, Literature, and Thought.* New York: Basic Books.

Searle, J. 2015. *Seeing Things as They Are: A Theory of Perception.* Oxford: Oxford University Press.

Stanghellini, G. 2004. *Disembodied Spirits and Deanimatied Bodies: The Psychopathology of Common Sense.* Oxford: Oxford University Press.

Straus, E. 1963. "Philosophische Grundlagen der Psychiatrie: Psychiatrie und Philosophie." In H. W. Gruhle, R. Jung, W. Mayer-Gross, M. Müller (eds.) *Psychiatrie der Gegenwart.* Bd. I/2. Berlin, Göttingen: Springer (pp. 926–994).

Thompson, E. 2007. *Mind in Life: Biology, Phenomenology, and the Sciences of Mind.* Cambridge, MA: Harvard University Press.

Tomasello, M. 1999. *The Cultural Origins of Human Cognition.* Cambridge, MA: Harvard University Press.

Tomasello, M., H. Rakoczy. 2003. "What makes human cognition unique? From individual to shared intentionality." *Mind & Language* **18**(2): 121–147.

Tomasello, M. 2019. *Becoming Human. A Theory of Ontogeny.* Cambridge/MA: Harvard University Press.

Uexküll, J. v. 2001. "An introduction to Umwelt." *Semiotica* **134**: 107–110.

Uexküll, J. v. 1973. *Theoretische Biologie.* Frankfurt/M.: Suhrkamp (1st ed. 1920).

Varela, F. J., E. Thompson, E. Rosch. 1991. *The Embodied Mind: Cognitive Science and Human Experience.* Cambridge, MA: MIT Press.

Vygotsky, L. S. 1978. *Mind in Society: Development of Higher Psychological Processes*. Trans. M. Cole. Cambridge, MA: Harvard University Press.

Weizsäcker, V. V. 1986. *Der Gestaltkreis. Theorie der Einheit von Wahrnehmen und Bewegen*. 5th ed. (1st ed. 1940). Stuttgart: Thieme.

Zahavi, D. 2001. *Husserl and Transcendental Intersubjectivity: A Response to the Linguistic-Pragmatic Critique*. Trans. Elizabeth A. Behnke. Ohio: Ohio University Press.

C

Psychiatry and Society

Chapter 8

Psychiatry between Psyche and Brain

Introduction

The British psychiatrist Sir Martin Roth once described psychiatry as "the most humane of the sciences and the most scientific of the humanities" (cf. Cawley 1993: 159). This aphorism expresses the hybrid character of psychiatry, but also its unique bridging position. Located between the natural sciences and the humanities, being theoretical and applied science in equal measure, focusing on human beings in their physical, psychological, and social existence—psychiatry thus probably has the widest range of the scientific disciplines. This range is both a burden and a task. It can lead to the formation of camps and to an increasing heterogeneity of the field, but also to an integration of aspects that can do justice to the complexity of the human being in a unique way. It can lead to recurring identity crises of the discipline, but it can also found its special identity and attractiveness.

Ever since its emergence around 1800, psychiatry has been operating in the tension between the humanities and natural sciences, between understanding and explanation, between psyche and brain. Over the last century, conflicts between biological, psychodynamic, anthropological, or social psychiatric approaches have continued to be fiercely fought out. Today, the transformation of psychiatry into a "clinical neuroscience" on a molecular biological basis appears to many as the overcoming of its changing history of errors and confusion (Insel & Quirion 2005). The traditional dualism of psyche and mind seems to dissolve into a neurobiological monism: "Mental disorders are brain disorders" is the guiding principle of biological psychiatry today (Insel & Quirion 2005; White et al. 2012).

Since the first "Decade of the Brain" from 1990 onwards, great hopes have been placed in this turnaround. As a scientific discipline, neuropsychiatry would soon be able to explain psychological diseases as brain dysfunctions and to diagnose them objectively with imaging procedures and other biomarkers. On this basis, it would be possible to develop highly specific medications and

In Defense of the Human Being. Thomas Fuchs, Oxford University Press. © Suhrkamp Verlag 2021.
DOI: 10.1093/oso/9780192898197.003.0009

even identify at-risk individuals for preventive treatment by means of genetic screening.[1]

The progress made since then in understanding the brain is indeed impressive. Whether one thinks of the identification of brain structures involved in numerous psychological functions as well as functional disorders such as anxiety, obsessive-compulsive or traumatic disorders, the epigenetic relationships of gene variants, life events, and vulnerability, or the knowledge about neuroplasticity and the influence of early socialization on brain development—there is no doubt that our understanding of the brain and its interactions with the environment has grown impressively.

And yet, after three decades, the result of brain research is sobering for psychiatry. Despite all the promises and billions of euros or dollars invested in research, hardly any clinically relevant findings have been brought to light. With the exception of Alzheimer's disease, there is no way to reliably diagnose psychiatric illnesses by means of instrumental examinations or biomarkers, or to assign them to specific gene variants (Cuthbert & Insel 2013). Nor have therapeutic procedures changed in any relevant way on the basis of neurobiological findings. All this is now acknowledged by high-ranking representatives of neurobiological research—to quote just a few of many examples:

> Despite obvious and rapid scientific advances, there is widespread frustration with the overall pace of progress in understanding and treating serious psychiatric illness. (Krystal & State 2014: 201)

> Unfortunately, there have been no major breakthroughs in the treatment of schizophrenia in the last 50 years and no major breakthroughs in the treatment of depression in the last 20 years. (Akil et al. 2010)

> Despite decades of research, the neurobiology of Major Depression is largely unknown, and treatments are no more effective today than they were 50–70 years ago. (Holtzheimer & Mayberg 2011: 1)

However, the usual consequence is not a reconsideration of the underlying reductionist paradigm, on the contrary. It is the traditional, fuzzy nosology and the outdated, subject-oriented psychopathology which are identified as the causes preventing the success of biological psychiatry (Cuthbert & Insel 2013; Krystal & State 2014). What is demanded is a completely new diagnostic approach, namely functional disorder domains (reward, attention, arousal, and other systems), which can be better classified according to molecular and

---

[1] Cf. Charney et al. (2002); Hyman (2003); Monyer et al. (2004); and Haag (2007).

imaging techniques.[2] In other medical disciplines, it is argued, molecular, imaging, and computer-based tools have also largely replaced clinical skills in diagnosis—why not in psychiatry (Jablensky& Kendell 2002)? This follows a well-known principle: what can be measured and grasped by technical means determines what is considered significant and finally regarded as actual reality. Such a research program may be perpetuated until the last convolution of the brain has been measured under special conditions of activity.

Now, the classical, subject-oriented psychopathology is certainly not set in stone. But already 10 years ago, Andreasen and other leading psychiatrists lamented the decline of psychopathological expertise as a result of criteriological diagnostic systems (Andreasen 2007; Mezzich 2007). The question arises whether psychiatry should run the risk of further losing this expertise, with the result that future psychiatrists know everything about reward systems in the brain but no longer know how to distinguish schizophrenia from hysteria. Moreover, it is by no means certain that mental illness can actually be broken down into the modular functions postulated by biological psychiatry. It seems much more probable that we are dealing with highly complex, mixed, context-related, and therefore inherently fuzzy processes (Nesse & Stein 2010; Sprevak 2011).

Despite all promises for "translational," i.e., application-oriented research, there is a risk that academic psychiatry's steps along this path increasingly separate it from clinical care and therapeutic practice—even as ever new "decades" of the brain, even the "century of the brain" are proclaimed, and new therapeutic breakthroughs announced.[3] Here, however, one usually refers to deep brain or magnetic stimulation, as the pharmaceutical industry has already largely withdrawn from research in the face of reduced chances of success (Abbott 2010; Miller 2010); even the much-vaunted "tailor-made" or "personalized psychiatry" based on individual bio-markers has remained a mere promise despite decades of research efforts (Perna et al. 2018). It is true that invasive brain therapy methods may be useful in extreme cases—but is this really the therapeutic prospect that neurobiological research opens up?

But perhaps we can stop at this point and ask ourselves: are we on the right track? Or are we losing sight of the phenomenon we are actually talking about—the psychological illness, the illness of a person—in the ever more focused, ultimately molecular biological view? Aren't the basic guiding assumptions,

---

[2] These are the so-called *Research Domain Criteria* developed by the National Institute of Mental Health in the USA (Cuthbert 2014; Carpenter 2016).

[3] "There is great promise for development of more effective treatments in the upcoming decade" (Insel 2014); see also Nature Editorial (2010).

"psyche = brain" and "mental illness = brain disease," too simple, perhaps not even true? In the following, I will examine these basic assumptions in order to present an alternative conception of psychiatry, namely as a *relational medicine* in a comprehensive sense.

Reductionist Assumptions and their Verification

Let us start again with the current demands of biological psychiatrists for a fundamental revision of our concepts of mental illness. Mental disorders are to be equated with functional disorders of brain circuits and thus, in essence, with neurological diseases (Insel & Wang 2010; White et al. 2012). In future, psychiatrists should call themselves "clinical neuroscientists," a change which would accelerate the integration of psychiatry into other medical disciplines and thus also contribute to the de-stigmatization of patients (Insel & Quirion 2005).[4] Such views are based on the reductionist assumption that subjective experiences such as feelings, desires, thoughts or intentions are ultimately only epiphenomena of brain processes. Psychological connections and explanations would then only be placeholders for molecular or neuronal causes yet to be discovered. The consequence would be a "psychiatry without psyche": mental illnesses would have nothing more to do with categories such as "meaning" or "interpretation" than strokes or other neurological failure syndromes.

But there are a whole range of objections to this view—I will mention only the most important ones:

(1) First of all, neural or genetic data only ever provide statistical deviations, not diagnoses. Brain states in themselves do not reveal what is considered healthy and what is Abnormal—only the clinic, i.e., the person suffering from mental illness, tells us this. However, the definition of mental illness is thus largely dependent on subjective and cultural factors that lie outside the realm of natural science (Kirmayer & Gold 2012). Therefore, the neuropsychiatrist is not only dependent on the patient's statements in his or her research, but also on a precise phenomenological analysis of these

---

[4] The latter hope has proved to be deceptive. Meta-analyses of numerous studies (Read et al. 2006; Schomerus et al. 2012) showed that although the biomedical concept of brain disease has become widespread among the general public over the last 20 years, it has never led to de-stigmatization—on the contrary: the majority of respondents perceive a mental disorder as strange, abnormal, or even threatening if it is based on a disorder of the genes or the brain rather than on psychosocial causes. And, the patients themselves can be relieved of feelings of guilt by a biological explanation, but at the cost of experiencing their symptoms and problems as fateful and beyond their control (Fuchs 2006).

statements. Without differentiated psychopathology, there can be no valid neurobiological research.

(2) Deviations from average brain activity do not, as such, indicate the cause of a disorder—it may just as well be a concomitant or consequence. The cause of a grief reaction is certainly not the activation of the cingulate cortex, which can be observed with it, but rather a loss experienced as painful. And it is not the activation of the amygdala that causes fear, but primarily the *subjective perception and evaluation* of a threatening situation—and this perception is not to be found in the amygdala, as necessary as it is as a substrate for the experience of fear. The bilateral *failure* of the amygdala certainly leads to fearlessness (Feinstein et al. 2011); but the *overreaction* of the amygdala in panic disorders is not their cause but rather a consequence of its physiological adaptation to repeated experiences of danger (LeDoux 1998). Of course, images suggest their own reality, and so neuroimaging all too easily leads to a confusion between *correlate* or substrate and *cause*. But the linear concept of causality of the nineteenth century—brain condition A produces disease B—does not allow us to understand the complex etiologies of mental disorders, even less so if we fail to take into account the *experience* of the patients in their life situation.

(3) This brings us to the central role of *subjectivity*, i.e., experience from the perspective of the first person. If we look at the triggering of depression, for example, it is usually based on the perception of a life situation as unmanageable and threatening—a perception that cannot be reduced to neuronal processes. However, this means that subjective, biographically acquired perceptual and behavioral dispositions gain crucial importance for pathogenesis, including self-concept, self-esteem, and self-efficacy (Fuchs 2012). The changed self-experience and self-relationship of the patient is also a constantly effective component in the *course* of the illness. It includes, for example, negative self-evaluations and depressive thought patterns, which in turn increase the probability of further failures and defeats. This leads to negative feedback and vicious circles, which exacerbate the depression. Without such circular processes a mental disorder cannot be adequately understood.

(4) If a mental illness cannot be detached from the person and attributed solely to the brain substrate, it can just as little be considered as a purely individual disorder, without its *interpersonal* aspect. Mental illnesses are caused by unfavorable life events and social influences, i.e., by disturbances in communication and relationship with others, and the resulting risk of illness is far higher than the genetic risk variable (van Os et al. 2008; Meyer-Lindenberg

& Tost 2012). Conversely, the illnesses impair the ability of patients to respond adequately to their social environment—with detrimental social consequences that in turn are decisive for the course of the illness. All these influences are undoubtedly mediated by neurobiological as well as epigenetic processes, but they are only taken up, not generated, by the brain.

In the last decade, social neuropsychiatry has made significant progress in researching the complex relationships between environmental influences, gene expression, brain structure, and disease disposition.[5] For example, it is now examining the influence of migration, urbanization, or social exclusion on the development of schizophrenia—which has admittedly long been known from epidemiological and social psychiatric studies (Read et al. 2009; Kirmayer & Gold 2012)—down to epigenetic and molecular micro processes. However, even these interrelationships have not yet revealed any possibilities for specific biological intervention, but they remain primarily the subject of social psychiatric action. Moreover, reductionist tendencies are also discernible here, since experience or interpersonal relationships hardly play a role in typical depictions, and the epigenetic mechanisms, which are mostly researched in animal experiments, are simply transferred to humans:

> Exploring the mechanisms of gene-environment interactions for depression is not substantially different from understanding how environmental toxins contribute to cancer or how diet influences cardiovascular disease. (Insel & Quirion 2005: 2221)

What is completely overlooked here is that it depends crucially on *subjective experience and evaluation* whether a stressor promotes resilience in one person but becomes a trauma in another, or how unemployment, separations, and social exclusion affect the psyche of a person, to name but a few examples. There is simply no direct effect of environmental factors on the brain—apart from a concussion. What permanently changes brain structures are the experiences that a person has in their social environment. But these experiences cannot be described as neurophysiological processes from the perspective of the third person, because they are bound to conscious experience, communication, and relationships.

To give an example, if a speaker's words leave an aftereffect in the brains of his audience, it is because he is speaking *to them*, not to their neurons and synapses, and because speaker and audience are jointly focused on words, meanings, and the objects they refer to. If the listeners were to fall asleep, this effect would soon be over, although the same stimuli would still reach their ears and brains. Joint attention, shared intentionality, experienced and practiced from

[5] Cf. for example, Akil et al. (2010); Heim & Binder (2012); Meyer-Lindenberg & Tost (2012).

childhood on—it is such overarching, conscious, and intentional experiences that leave traces in our brains, not a flow of physical stimuli or data from a mouth to a brain.

Mere data streams have no meaning whatsoever as long as there are no subjects for whom something like significance and meaning emerge in the first place. In meanings we refer to something in the world, they are *relations*, and these do not exist inside the head. Therefore, our conscious experiences are not just epiphenomena of neurophysiological processes. Rather, the opposite is true: the neuronal processes in our brains are only *parts or components* of overarching psychological, i.e., subjective and intersubjective processes. And, if psychotherapies demonstrably change the function and structure of the brain (Fuchs 2004; Goldapple et al. 2004), then this is only because they consist of relational and intentional experiences, i.e., of meaningful processes and order patterns in which the brain is involved and by which it is changed—"top down," as they say. The *sharing* of feelings, words, and thoughts is what constitutes the healing therapeutic relationship. Subjectivity is a reality, it changes brains, it even changes the world.

This does not mean that the psyche becomes a free-floating substance that acts on the body or brain from outside, as it were. Rather, we refer to the psyche as *the overall gestalt, the form of appearance and the order patterns of all the relationships* we have as living beings to the environment and as human beings to other human beings. These forms of relationships are of course also realized through neuronal processes, but they can by no means be reduced to them. The psyche is not a hidden interior space produced in the brain. It is alive and embodied, it embraces the entire body as a sounding board for all feelings (Fuchs & Koch 2014); and at the same time it is our relationship to the world—be it the perception and handling of things or the emotion and communication with other people. None of this is to be found in the brain as such—brains see nothing, feel nothing, and think nothing, as indispensable as they are as *mediating* or "relational organs" for these overarching processes (Fuchs 2011).

Conscious experience therefore only arises in the comprehensive, ecological system of organism and environment, in the interplay of many components, to which the brain and the body with its entire inner milieu, with its senses and limbs, belong, just as much as the appropriate objects of the environment. Even the simple feat of catching an approaching ball cannot therefore be captured by brain research (Sprevak 2011), even less so the complex physical and verbal interactions that take place between two people.

The brain is undoubtedly the organ that mediates all these interactions—and which, due to its plasticity, is constantly modifying and structuring itself through interactions. It is an interactive, mediating organ. But, in the brain itself there is no experience, no consciousness, no thoughts—all this exists only in the interplay of organism and environment. It is relationships and interactions that form our psyche and our brain from birth, that create our experience and our common world, and that give substance and meaning to our life. And, when we learn today that even an organic disease such as Alzheimer's dementia can best be prevented through physical movement and social interaction (Rolland et al. 2008; Pillai & Verghese 2009), this shows all the more that we have to understand the brain as an organ of relationships—as an organ of the psyche, not as a supposedly localizable inner world, but rather of the psyche as a comprehensive, embodied, and interactive life process.

A discipline that carries the psyche in its name cannot therefore be limited to the analysis of molecules, genes, and neurons. Molecular and neuronal processes, as well as their deviations or dysfunctions, are only parts of higher-level circular processes in which psychic life consists. Imaging does not provide a view of the psyche either, but only the visualization of necessary partial functions—just as the oxygen concentration in the pulmonary alveoli only represents one component of breathing, but not the overall exchange between the organism and the environment in which breathing actually exists.

Just like breathing through the lungs, all mental exchange processes take place through the brain. Nevertheless, very different biological, psychological, and social influences can contribute to their disorders. However, if mental illnesses do not affect the brain alone but the interaction between brain, organization, and environment, it is no longer surprising that brain scans do not adequately capture the underlying pathology (Banner 2013). Because in these interactions, it is precisely that which is systematically dismissed in a purely scientific approach that plays the decisive role: subjectivity and intersubjectivity. The fact *that they are experienced and take place in relationships* makes psychological processes and psychological disorders so complex that they cannot be represented in mere neurological sub-functions.

Psychiatry as Relational Medicine: An Integrative Concept

It seems to be time to look for a new conception of psychiatry that leaves behind the classical dualism of body and psyche as well as its neuro-reductionist alternative. Such an integrative concept should enable us to understand the overarching ecological contexts in which mental illnesses develop and how biological, psycho-, and socio-therapeutic treatment approaches intertwine. However, the "biopsysocial model" (Engel 1977) often referred to involves a compromise solution and is content with a mere juxtaposition of causal factors

(Ghaemi 2009). Today, it can be replaced by concepts of dynamic circular processes, such as those already developed in the *functional circle* of von Uexküll (1920/1973) or the *gestalt circle* of von Weizsäcker (1940/1986). Whether we look at the relationships between brain and body, between organization and environment, or the relationships between people, they all consist in circular feedback interactions.

In the current concepts of embodied and enactive cognition (Varela et al. 1991; Thompson 2007; Drayson 2009), psychiatry could also find an expanded paradigm that understands the brain, organism and environment in their dynamic unity. Neuronal processes become components of a comprehensive process that can be viewed on different levels: the *macro-level* of psychosocial processes or the interactions of persons, the *medium, individual level* of interactions between brain, organism and environment, and the *micro-level* of neuronal and molecular processes within the brain. Descending to the next level, the selected section of the event narrows. However, the levels cannot be reduced to one another; there is instead a relationship of emergence between them (see Fig. 8.1).

This leads to both top-down and bottom-up effects. A psychotherapeutic treatment as an interactive, intentional process on the macro level modifies the brain structures involved—*top-down*. The altered neuronal structure, however, in turn enables the patient's interactions with the environment to change—*bottom-up*, and so on. In the course of time, a mutual influence of superordinate psychosocial interactions and neuronal substrate, or of *process* and *structure*, develops (Fuchs 2018: 139–140). Biological, psycho-, and socio-therapeutic interventions start at different levels and components, but they are interlinked in circles and can also be used to complement each other: it is only important that the circular processes receive a new direction through the therapeutic impulse.

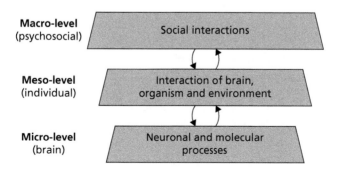

Fig. 8.1 Levels of embodied interactions with top-down and bottom-up relations (↓↑)

From this point of view, mental disorders are always disorders of the *overarching* processes at the macro-level, i.e., they affect the patients in their self-awareness and relationships. However, individuals are also living, embodied beings and all their psychological processes are also biological processes—not limited to the brain, of course. Above all, a correctly understood biological psychiatry requires an adequate concept of *biology*, namely that of life bound to the entire organism and its interaction with the environment. It requires an *ecological theory* that includes social and cultural processes outside the brain, even if they are functionally reflected in genome and brain structures. Only then can it correctly understand the brain as the central mediating organ for these superordinate processes; only then can social neuroscience contribute important components to understanding the mechanisms involved (Schilbach et al. 2013; Kotchoubey et al. 2016).

To proclaim psychiatry only as clinical neuroscience or to expect salvation from "genomics" and "proteomics" would be mistaken. After all, the experience and relationships of the patient are at the core of mental illness, and they cannot be identified with neuronal or molecular processes. Instead, we should understand psychiatry as a *comprehensive relational medicine*: as the *science and practice of biological, psychological and social relationships and their disorders*. An ecological concept of the psyche as the overarching form of the relations between organism and environment, between person and world, would be suitable to substantiate such a relational medicine. Without doubt, all the biological processes involved belong to the terrain of this psychiatry. At its center, however, is the *person* in his or her relationship to other people, because it is in the patient himself or herself that all the levels and circular processes that we observe, which we can explore and in which we can also intervene, unite.

Conclusion

A person-centered psychiatry will always see more in mental illness than just brain disease. The patients' experience and relationship to themselves and others are the central components of the illness. For this reason, the description or imaging of neuronal processes only ever reveals part of the overall disease process, even if neuronal dysfunctions play a major role in the pathogenesis and may be the starting point for significant therapeutic procedures. However, no psychiatric illness can be diagnosed, described, or treated without considering the patient's subjectivity and interpersonal relationships. Mental illnesses always affect the person in their relationship with others.

Under this premise, the research efforts of the discipline must be equally focused on biological processes, psychopathological experiences, psychological-biographical connections, and social interactions, instead of being reduced to analyzing processes inside the brain. The question of an adequate use and distribution of financial resources must then also be asked in research, not only in medical care. Last but not least, psychiatry should also reflect on its person-oriented traditions. A psychiatry of the person will undoubtedly also give individual genetics and neurobiology their appropriate place in a comprehensive diagnostics and therapy. However, the relationship between psychiatrist and patient remains of paramount importance, since, as the American psychiatrist John Nemiah once put it:

> […] we are ourselves the instrument that sounds the depth of the patient's being, reverberates with his emotions, detects his hidden conflicts, and perceives the gestalt of his recurring patterns of behavior. (Nemiah 1989)

No brain scan, no matter how much detail it reveals, could ever be superior to this instrument. This is the core of the psychiatric profession, and it is also what patients genuinely expect from their psychiatrists: they want to be understood and share their experiences with them. They want to be recognized, acknowledged and accompanied, especially in their self-alienation and confusion.

But the ability to do so is an *art*. It must be trained, educated, supported by suitable instruments of phenomenological assessment,[6] and above all taught by role models, because it cannot be represented in diagnostic algorithms. A subject-oriented, understanding psychopathology is still indispensable for a valid diagnosis (Fuchs 2010). At the same time, it establishes the primary therapeutic relationship to the patient. In combination with a careful anamnesis, behavior or conflict analysis, it becomes the starting point for any treatment, and this will in each case only be successful if it is embedded in a trusting relationship. The therapeutic alliance has consistently proven to be the decisive factor for a positive course of treatment of psychotherapies (Martin et al. 2000); similarly, adherence, placebo effect, and the success of a pharmacotherapy depend significantly on the therapeutic alliance.[7]

It is in the understanding and therapeutic relationship with the patient that the real wealth of the discipline lies, the real psychiatric art, and it is ultimately this that distinguishes it fundamentally from primarily organic disciplines such as neurology. If psychiatry sees itself as relational medicine, it can become the forerunner of a development that is important for the future of medicine as a whole, namely a medicine of the person in their biological, psychological, and

---

[6] See for example Parnas et al. (2005) or Sass et al. (2017).

[7] On this, cf. Frank & Gunderson (1990), Krupnick et al. (1996), Weiss et al. (1997), McCabe & Priebe (2004), Stavropoulou (2011).

ecological relationships. It is precisely because of the complexity of their discipline that psychiatrists are in a position to mediate between natural sciences and humanities, between objective and subject-oriented, individual and social aspects, and to develop integrative perspectives. Psychiatrists should therefore not deny the tense, often conflictual identity of their field. On the contrary, they should defend it with self-confidence and conviction, because it is a deeply humane identity. Its primary object is not the brain, but the person living in relationships.

References

Abbott, A. 2010. "The drug deadlock." *Nature* **468**(7321): 158–159.

Akil, H., S. Brenner, E. Kandel, K. S. Kendler, M. C. King, E. Scolnick, J. D. Watson, H. Y. Zoghbi. 2010. "The future of psychiatric research: Genomes and neural circuits." *Science* **327**(5973): 1580–1581.

Andreasen, N. C. 2007. "DSM and the death of phenomenology in America: An example of unintended consequences." *Schizophrenia Bulletin* **33**(1): 108–112.

Banner, N. F. 2013. "Mental disorders are not brain disorders." *Journal of Evaluation in Clinical Practice* **19**(3): 509–513.

Carpenter, W. T. 2016. "The RDoC controversy: Alternate paradigm or dominant paradigm?" *The American Journal of Psychiatry* **173**(6): 562–563.

Cawley, R. H. 1993. "Psychiatry is more than a science." *British Journal of Psychiatry* **162**: 154–160.

Charney, D. S., D. H. Barlow, K. Botteron, J. D. Cohen, D. Goldman, R. E. Gur, K.-M. Lin, J. F. López, J. H. Meador-Woodruff, S. O. Moldin, S. J. Zalcman. 2002. "Neuroscience research agenda to guide development of a pathophysiologically based classification system." In D. J. Kupfer, M. B. First, A. Regier (eds.) *A Research Agenda for DSM-V.* Arlington: American Psychiatric Association (pp. 31–83).

Cuthbert, B. N. 2014. "The RDoC framework: Facilitating transition from ICD/DSM to dimensional approaches that integrate neuroscience and psychopathology." *World Psychiatry* **13**(1): 28–35.

Cuthbert B. N., T. R. Insel. 2013. "Toward the future of psychiatric diagnosis: The seven pillars of RdoC." *BMC Medicine* **11**: Artikel 126. https://doi.org/10.1186/1741-7015-11-126, accessed on 03.12.2019.

Drayson, Z. 2009. "Embodied Cognitive Science and its Implications for Psychopathology." *Philosophy, Psychiatry, & Psychology* 16: 329–340.

Engel, G. 1977. "The need for a new medical model: A challenge for biomedicine." *Science* **196**(4286): 9–135.

Feinstein, J. S., R. Adolphs, A. Damasio, D. Tranel. 2011. "The human amygdala and the induction and experience of fear." *Current Biology* **21**(1): 34–38.

Frank, A. F., J. G. Gunderson. 1990. "The role of the therapeutic alliance in the treatment of schizophrenia: Relationship to course and outcome." *Archives of General Psychiatry* **47**(3): 228–236.

Fuchs, T. 2004. "Neurobiology and psychotherapy: An emerging dialogue." *Current Opinions in Psychiatry* **17**: 479–485.

Fuchs, T. 2006. "Ethical issues in neuroscience." *Current Opinions in Psychiatry* **19**(6): 600–607.

Fuchs, T. 2010. "Subjectivity and intersubjectivity in psychiatric diagnosis." *Psychopathology* **43**(4): 268–274.

Fuchs, T. 2011. "The brain—a mediating organ." *Journal of Consciousness Studies* **18**(7–8): 196–221.

Fuchs, T. 2012. "Are mental illnesses diseases of the brain?" In **S. Choudhury, S. K. Nagel, J. Slaby** (eds.) *Critical Neuroscience.* London: Wiley-Blackwell (pp. 331–344).

Fuchs, T. 2013. "The phenomenology and development of social perspectives." *Phenomenology and the Cognitive Sciences* **12**(4): 655–683.

Fuchs, T. 2018. *Ecology of the Brain: The Phenomenology and Biology of the Embodied Mind.* Oxford: Oxford University Press.

Fuchs, T., S. Koch. 2014. "Embodied affectivity: On moving and being moved." *Frontiers in Psychology* **5**: 508.

Ghaemi, N. 2009. "The rise and fall of the biopsychosocial model." *The British Journal of Psychiatry* **195**(1): 3–4.

Goldapple, K., Z. Segal, C. Garson, M. Lau, P. Bieling, S. Kennedy, H. Mayberg. 2004. "Modulation of cortical-limbic pathways in major depression. Treatment-specific effects of cognitive behavior therapy." *Archives of General Psychiatry* **61**(1): 34–41.

Griesinger, W. 1845. *Die Pathologie und Therapie der psychischen Krankheiten für Ärzte und Studirende.* Stuttgart: Adolph Krabbe.

Haag, A. 2007. "Biomarkers trump behavior in mental illness diagnosis." *Nature Medicine* **13**(1): 3–4.

Heim, C., E. B. Binder. 2012. "Current research trends in early life stress and depression: Review of human studies on sensitive periods, gene-environment interactions, and epigenetics." *Experimental Neurology* **233**(1): 102–111.

Holtzheimer, P. E., H. S. Mayberg. 2011. "Stuck in a rut: Rethinking depression and its treatment." *Trends in Neurosciences* **34**(1): 1–9.

Hyman, S. E. 2003. "Diagnosing disorders." *Scientific American* **289**(3): 96–103.

Insel, T. R. 2014. "Understanding mental disorders as circuit disorders." Online at: *BrainFacts. org* https://www.brainfacts.org/archives/2010/understanding-mental-disorders-as-circuit-disorders, accessed 01.06.2021.

Insel, T. R., R. Quirion. 2005. "Psychiatry as a clinical neuroscience discipline." *JAMA* **294**(17): 2221–2224.

Insel, T. R., P. S. Wang. 2010. "Rethinking mental illness." *JAMA* **303**(19): 1970–1971.

Jablensky, A., R. E. Kendell. 2002. "Criteria for assessing a classification in psychiatry." In **M. Maj, W. Gaebel, J. J. López-Ibor, N. Sartorius** (eds.) *Psychiatric Diagnosis and Classification.* Chichester: Wiley (pp. 1–25).

Kirmayer, L. J., I. Gold. 2012. "Re-socializing psychiatry." In **S. Choudhury, S. K. Nagel, J. Slaby** (eds.) *Critical Neuroscience.* London: Wiley-Blackwell (pp. 305–330).

Kotchoubey, B., F. Tretter, H. A. Braun, T. Buchheim, A. Draguhn, T. Fuchs, F. Hasler, H. Hastedt, T. Hinterberger, G. Northoff, I. Rentschler, S. Schleim, S. Sellmaier, L.

Tebartz van Elst, W. Tschacher. 2016. "Methodological problems on the way to integrative human neuroscience." *Frontiers in Integrative Neuroscience* **10**: 41.

Krupnick, J. L., S. M. Sotsky, S. Simmens, J. Moyer, I. Elkin, J. Watkins, P. A. Pilkonis. 1996. "The role of the therapeutic alliance in psychotherapy and pharmacotherapy outcome: Findings in the National Institute of Mental Health Treatment of Depression Collaborative Research Program." *Journal of Consulting and Clinical Psychology* **64**(3): 532–539.

Krystal, J. H., M. W. State. 2014. "Psychiatric disorders: Diagnosis to therapy." *Cell* **157**(1): 201–214.

LeDoux, J. 1998. "Fear and the brain: Where have we been, and where are we going?" *Biological Psychiatry* **44**(12): 1229–1238.

Martin, D. J., J. P. Garske, M. K. Davis. 2000. "Relation of the therapeutic alliance with outcome and other variables: A meta-analytic review." *Journal of Consulting and Clinical Psychology* **68**(3): 438–450.

McCabe, R., S. Priebe. 2004. "The therapeutic relationship in the treatment of severe mental illness: A review of methods and findings." *International Journal of Social Psychiatry* **50**(2): 115–128.

Meyer-Lindenberg, A., H. Tost. 2012. "Neural mechanisms of social risk for psychiatric disorders." *Nature Neuroscience* **15**(5): 663–668.

Mezzich, J. E. 2007. "Psychiatry for the person: Articulating medicine's science and humanism." *World Psychiatry* **6**(2): 65–67.

Miller, G. 2010. Is pharma running out of brainy ideas?' *Science* **329**(5991): 502–504.

Monyer, H., F. Rösler, G. Roth, H. Scheich, W. Singer, C. E. Elger, A. D. Friederici, C. Koch, H. Luhmann, C. von der Malsburg, R. Menzel. 2004. "Das Manifest. Elf führende Neurowissenschaftler über Gegenwart und Zukunft der Hirnforschung." *Gehirn und Geist* (6): 30–37.

Nature Editorial. 2010. "A decade for psychiatric disorders." *Nature* **463**(7277): 9.

Nemiah, J. C. 1989. "The varieties of human experience." *The British Journal of Psychiatry* **154**: 459–466.

Nesse, R. M., D. J. Stein. 2010. "Towards a genuinely medical model for psychiatric nosology." *BMC Medicine* **10**: Artikel 5. https://doi.org/10.1186/1741-7015-10-5, accessed 04.12.2019.

Parnas, J., P. Møller, T. Kircher, J. Thalbitzer, L. Jansson, P. Handest, D. Zahavi. 2005. "EASE: Examination of anomalous self-experience." *Psychopathology* **38**(5): 236–258.

Perna, G., M. Grassi, D. Caldirola, C. B. Nemeroff. 2018. "The revolution of personalized psychiatry: will technology make it happen sooner?" *Psychological Medicine* **48**(5): 705–713.

Pillai, J. A., J. Verghese. 2009. "Social networks and their role in preventing dementia." *Indian Journal of Psychiatry* **51**(Supplement 1): 22–28.

Read, J., R. P. Bentall, R. Fosse. 2009. "Time to abandon the bio-bio-bio model of psychosis: Exploring the epigenetic and psychological mechanisms by which adverse life events lead to psychotic symptoms." *Epidemiology and Psychiatric Sciences* **18**(4): 299–310.

Read, J., N. Haslam, L. Sayce, E. Davies. 2006. "Prejudice and schizophrenia: A review of the 'mental illness is an illness like any other' approach." *Acta Psychiatrica Scandinavica* **114**(5): 303–318.

Rolland, Y., G. A. van Kan, B. Vellas. 2008. "Physical activity and Alzheimer's disease: From prevention to therapeutic perspectives." *Journal of the American Medical Directors Association* 9(6): 390–405.

Sass, L., E. Pienkos, B. Škodlar, G. Stanghellini, T. Fuchs, J. Parnas, N. Jones. 2017. "EAWE: Examination of anomalous world experience." *Psychopathology* 50(1): 10–54.

Schilbach, L., B. Timmermans, V. Reddy, A. Costall, G. Bente, T. Schlicht, K. Vogeley. 2013. "Toward a second-person neuroscience." *The Behavioral and Brain Sciences* 36(4): 393–414.

Schomerus, G., C. Schwahn, A. Holzinger, P. W. Corrigan, H. J. Grabe, M. G. Carta, M. C. Angermeyer. 2012. "Evolution of public attitudes about mental illness: A systematic review and meta-analysis." *Acta Psychiatrica Scandinavica* 125(6): 440–452.

Sprevak, M. 2011. "Neural sufficiency, reductionism, and cognitive neuropsychiatry." *Philosophy, Psychiatry, & Psychology* 18(4): 339–344.

Stavropoulou, C. 2011. "Non-adherence to medication and doctor–patient relationship: Evidence from a European survey." *Patient Education and Counseling* 83(1): 7–13.

Thompson, E. 2007. *Mind in Life: Biology, Phenomenology, and the Sciences of Mind.* Cambridge, MA: Harvard University Press.

Uexküll, J. V. 1973. *Theoretische Biologie.* Frankfurt/M.: Suhrkamp. (First published 1920.)

van Os, J., B. P. Rutten, R. Poulton. 2008. "Gene-environment interactions in schizophrenia: Review of epidemiological findings and future directions." *Schizophrenia Bulletin* 34(6): 1066–1082.

Varela, F. J., E. Thompson, E. Rosch 1991. *The Embodied Mind: Cognitive Science and Human Experience.* Cambridge, MA: MIT Press.

Weiss, M., L. Gaston, A. Propst, S. Wisebord, V. Zicherman. 1997. "The role of the alliance in the pharmacologic treatment of depression." *Journal of Clinical Psychiatry* 58(5): 196–204.

Weizsäcker, V. V. 1986. *Der Gestaltkreis: Theorie der Einheit von Wahrnehmen und Bewegen.* Stuttgart: Thieme (Originally published 1940.)

White, P. D., H. Rickards, A. Z. J. Zeman. 2012. "Time to end the distinction between mental and neurological illnesses." *British Medical Journal* 344: e3454.

Chapter 9

Embodiment and Personal Identity in Dementia

Introduction

"I have, so to speak, lost myself"—this was the complaint of Auguste Deter, the first patient diagnosed by Alois Alzheimer in 1901 with the illness that was later named after him (Maurer et al. 1997). Alzheimer's disease and other dementias seem particularly unsettling and threatening, as they call into question that which we perceive as the foundation of being ourselves: our cognitive and reflective capacities. To be a person in the full sense of the word is, in Western cultures, decisively bound up with the intactness of functions such as reflection, rationality, memory, and with the autonomy that is based on them. Impairments resulting from a process of dementia therefore come into conflict with the central values of a culture centered on cognition and on the individual. Dementia becomes a threat to the person as such and is more stigmatized than most other mental illnesses: in the advanced stages, the loss of rationality and autobiographical memory appears to leave behind only a bodily facade, the utterances of which allow the recognition of mere fragments of the earlier person. For ethical utilitarians such as Singer (1979) or McMahan (2003), people with severe dementia appear consequentially no longer to be persons as such, but rather to be "quasi-persons" or "post-persons" (McMahan 2003: 46 ff., 55).

However, this identification of our selfhood with cognition, rationality, and memory is based on a dualistic conception of personhood, in which the body serves merely as a vehicle for the mind—or the brain. According to this view, the cortex and the act of thinking become the site of the person, while the rest of the body, along with our embodied feelings, lacks cognitive awareness and rational control and so leads nothing more than a shadow existence. Such a view, I argue, neglects what is constitutive of human personhood, namely its sociality, which already manifests itself in the primary, pre-reflective intersubjectivity of early childhood, and which is crucially based on intercorporeality and interaffectivity (Stern 1985; Trevarthen 1993; Fuchs 2017a).

In this chapter, I will counter the cognitivist perspective on dementia with another conception of personhood, which has its foundation in the

In Defense of the Human Being. Thomas Fuchs, Oxford University Press. © Suhrkamp Verlag 2021.
DOI: 10.1093/oso/9780192898197.003.0010

phenomenology of the body. Here, our primary selfhood is essentially vital and bodily. Only as a body can a human sense and express itself, and encounter other humans and the world. Everything to do with perception, thought, and action is performed through the medium of the body: the eyes see, the ears hear, the hands hold, and the tongue speaks, all without our direct awareness. Whatever we consciously plan or do, we proceed from a bodily foundation which we are never able to make fully conscious to ourselves. This foundation, as I will show, is never completely lost, even in dementia. Moreover, it also forms the basis of an intercorporeality that always already connects us with others, without requiring explicit, symbolically mediated interaction.

The subjective or lived body also has its own history. From early childhood, its experiences have sedimented as sensorimotor habits and capabilities of dealing with objects and other people. All of these habits and experiences can be brought together in the term "body memory." This points towards a continuity of the person which is not rooted in in a repertoire of memories but rather in experience sedimented in the body. It is only recently that this form of memory has been taken into account for understanding and treating dementia.[1] And, indeed, it is a kind of memory which remains preserved right up to the last stages of the illness, and in which the biographical history of the patient is manifested.

In what follows, I first consider personal identity from a cognitivist and then from an embodied perspective, before focusing on the role of body memory for the continuity of the self. Turning to dementia, I first describe it as a loss of reflexivity and meta-perspective, which I then contrast with the preservation of body memory and intercorporeality. This will allow me to argue for the continuity of the pre-reflective self even in late stages of the illness. A final look will be given to narrativistic and constructionist concepts of the self in dementia which I contrast with an embodied notion of personhood.

Personal Identity

The cognitivist conception of person has a history which goes back to the origins of European modernity and which is characterized by the growing separation of the personal subject from its corporeality and vitality. The dualistic and rationalistic understanding of person in the work of Descartes or Locke is bound up with self-consciousness, cognition, and rational reflection, as the modern subject wants to be certain of itself, sovereign and autonomous. However, this certitude of the cogito is only ever possible as an instantaneous

---

[1] See Kontos (2004); Fleischman et al. (2005); Golby et al. (2005), and Harrison et al. (2007).

self-consciousness. No longer embedded in its corporeality, the Ego must continuously think in order to exist, and reflect upon itself, in order to be certain of itself. Yet what does the res cogitans, that thinking thing, do when it does not think, when it has to surrender to the body, to sleep or forgetting? What is it then that enables the lasting continuity of the person? Early on, Locke identified this as a problem with the Cartesian subject:

> But that which seems to make the difficulty, is this, that this consciousness being interrupted always by forgetfulness […] in all these cases […] doubts are raised whether we are the same thinking thing; i.e. the same substance or no. (Locke: Essay II, xxvii; cf. Locke 1997: 302–3)

Locke's solution, which has remained influential until today, was the following: it is self-consciousness and memory which allows a person to extend himself into time beyond the present:

> For as far as any intelligent being can repeat the idea of any past action, and with the same consciousness it has of any present action; so far it is the same personal self. (Locke 1997: 303)

Memory thus builds the necessary bridge: the unity and identity of the person is bound to the possibility of conscious remembering. With its help, past episodes are assimilated and integrated in the present self. This means, however, that I remain myself only so long as I can recall my previous states and accredit them to myself. Locke's view continues to this day in the psychological conception of personal persistence:[2] the identity of a person reaches only as far as his memory of himself remains intact. Yet, this view has the counterintuitive consequence that we can strictly speaking neither ascribe states of sleep nor our fetal and infant states to ourselves because these are not states we can remember. Moreover, if patients in schizophrenia are delusional and consider themselves another person, they would lose their personhood for the duration of the delusion. The same would apply to patients with advanced dementia who can no longer remember their previous experiences.

But in which way is the self lost in dementia? Is it really the case that our selfhood, our identity, depends solely on our memory and knowledge of ourselves? By no means, because this knowledge of the "self-as-object" is preceded by the "self-as-subject," a continual, pre-reflective experience of self which does not need to be made explicit or grasped in words. For most of our daily lives we do not make ourselves conscious of who we are, do not reflect on ourselves, or recall autobiographical memories—we are just aware of ourselves as a matter

---

[2] Principal representatives are, for example, Shoemaker (1970), Parfit (1984), or Garrett (1998).

of course (Klein 2013; Fuchs 2017b). There is no need for being reflectively self-conscious, remembering the past, or other forms of explicit psychological connectedness which Lockeans have in mind. Moreover, in our first moments of awakening from sleep, we already find ourselves in our basic bodily sense of self, prior to any memory of the day before, even less of our biography. Reflective self-consciousness is a possibility, but not a necessary condition of being one-self. We could persist as selves with pre-reflective self-awareness, based on the background feeling of the body, even though this is normally superimposed by multiple facets of self-reflection, self-knowledge, and memories, or in other words, by the self-as-object. So when Auguste Deter complained "I have lost myself," she obviously still had a sense of self, otherwise her sentence would not have had a subject. What she had lost was the self-as-object, or her knowledge about herself, not the self-as-subject.

As Locke did not distinguish between reflective and pre-reflective self-experience, he could only base the sense of identity on recollection. However, the lived body conveys a continuity of selfhood, which ultimately represents the subjective side of the life process itself and does not require reflective self-identification. In this sense, Merleau-Ponty described the lived body as the "natural subject," which is the precedent and foundation for all conscious and reflective acts. Were we to be without this basal experience of self, then all bio-graphical knowledge would be useless to us, as our self would be lost in an elementary sense, and there would be no one to ascribe this knowledge to. As meaningful as the possible grasp of this knowledge might be for our narrative identity, selfhood in a foundational sense is not bound to biographical memory nor to knowledge about oneself. It is rather an intrinsic quality of every experience, a self-givenness of the continuous stream of consciousness as such (Zahavi 1999, 2006). As we will see, such a basal self-experience remains intact even in late stages of dementia.

The phenomenology of the bodily subject can be expanded to a conception of embodied personhood which integrates the aspect of the lived body (*Leib*) and the aspect of the living body or organism (*Körper*). This can only be outlined briefly here (for an extensive depiction see Fuchs 2017b, 2018). According to the paradigm of embodied cognition, consciousness is not a pure product of the brain, but is rather a comprehensive activity of the entire organism in relation to its environment. Only a brain connected to a sensory, perceptive, and moveable body is in a position to serve as an operating organ for psychological processes; the reason for this is that it is only through the continuous interaction between brain, body, and environment that the forms of conscious experience emerge and stabilize themselves. In this respect, personhood is a manifestation of the life process of a human organism and it is thereby embodied in the capabilities and activities of the whole body. Moreover, we are also embodied persons for each other: we do not perceive a body-object whose movements lead us to infer an "inhabitant" hidden in the brain like in a capsule. Rather, the lived body itself is the living appearance and expression of the person "in the flesh."

Body Memory

As we have seen, the assurance of being-with-oneself, which the Cartesian subject believed to have found in self-observation and memory, always precedes these reflective acts. Now, one could object that this pre-reflective self-awareness only concerns a "minimal self" (Zahavi 2006) which barely satisfies our expectations of individuality and personhood. Bodily existence would give us just an anonymous identity or sameness but no qualitative identity—being the sort of persons that we are. In order to adequately evaluate the significance of pre-reflective self-awareness for personal continuity, we have to further explore the temporality of this layer of experience.

First, we are dealing here not with an instantaneous but an extended and continuous self-experience, which is based on the unfolding and connection of protentions, impressions, and retentions as analyzed by Husserl (1991). It is this connection which establishes the ongoing continuity of the pre-reflective self (Zahavi 1999: 73). This continuity is not restricted to fleeting experiences, however. It extends over the entire life span, once we consider the history of the lived body, which, in the course of a biography, becomes ever more a medium of our individual existence. All performances of life enter into the memory of the body and remain preserved as dispositions and potentialities: as Merleau-Ponty pointed out, the body is "solidified existence" and, for its part, "existence [is] perpetual incarnation" (Merleau-Ponty 1962: 148). Let us consider this history of the body in more detail.

The explicit or autobiographical memory with which Locke was concerned is by no means the only form of continuity which establishes itself over the course of our life. The majority of that which we have experienced and learned does not become accessible to us in retrospect, but far more in the practical movements of everyday life: habits are built up through repetition and practice and they are activated by themselves; established processes of movement are merged "into our flesh and blood"—such as walking upright, speaking, or writing, dealing with objects such as a bicycle or a piano. We can designate the totality of sedimented experiences the *implicit* or *body memory*.[3] Already conceived in the

---

[3] On this, see Casey 1984; Schacter 1987; and Fuchs 2011, 2012. In the cognitive and neuro-psychological literature, the term implicit memory usually comprises procedural memory,

work of Maine de Biran (1953) and Henri Bergson (1988), body memory envisions the past not in retrospect, but preserves it as accumulated and currently effective experience. It is actualized through the medium of the body without requiring us to recall earlier situations, or in other words, it is our lived past.

This body memory emerges in different types (Fuchs 2012), four of which I wish to sketch briefly:

1) As *procedural memory*, we may designate the already mentioned sensorimotor capabilities of the body: well-practiced habits, the skillful handling of tools and instruments as well as familiarity with patterns of perception, acquired through repetition and practice. This memory relieves our attention from an overflow of details and enables the unreflective activities of everyday life. It facilitates the kind of action in which we turn our attention to the goal of the performance rather than each individual movement; for example, the melody we wish to play with an instrument, and not the separate movements of our fingers.

2) *Situational body memory* enables us to recognize familiar situations and to skillfully cope with them. This concerns in particular spatial situations in which we find our bearings, such as in an apartment, in a neighborhood, or in a hometown. Bodily experiences connect particularly to interior spaces, and the more often this happens, the more the room is filled with a familiar, intimate atmosphere. "Inhabiting" and "habit" are equally grounded in body memory. The following example from Gaston Bachelard demonstrates this:

> But over and beyond our memories, the house we were born in is physically inscribed in us. It is a group of organic habits. After twenty years, in spite of all the other anonymous stairways; we would recapture the reflexes of the "first stairway," we would not stumble on that rather high step. The house's entire being would open up, faithful to our own being [...] The word habit is too worn a word to express this passionate liaison of our bodies, which do not forget, with an unforgettable house. (Bachelard: 1964, 92f.)

In this way, through its situational memory, the body connects with complementary environmental affordances (Gibson 1979) or "offerings"—things being graspable, viable, attractive, repulsive, etc., in accordance with already acquired experience and skills.

---

skill learning, and priming effects (Schacter 1987, 1996). However, I use the term interchangeably with "body memory" in an extended sense which also covers types of embodied memory such as intercorporeal, emotional, pain, or traumatic memory (see following section). By contrast, the explicit memory system, also termed "declarative memory," includes autobiographical or episodic memory and semantic knowledge.

3) Intuitive, non-verbal communication with others, including the empathic understanding of their expressions, is also based on acquired capacities of the body, namely on the *intercorporeal memory*, which goes back as far as earliest childhood. In the first year of life, infants already learn patterns of social interactions with others which imprint themselves in their body long before the development of biographical memory, which occurs in the second year of life. In infant research, one speaks of implicit relational knowledge (Stern 1998)—how one shares pleasure with others, shows joy, avoids rejection, and so forth. We find another form of intercorporeal memory in well-coordinated dance partners who move easily with the rhythm of the music, and their hands and bodies interact without the need of any verbal or visual guidance.

4) Finally, body memory also includes those individual habits, attitudes and roles that have often been taken over from others and have been incorporated as an embodied personality structure; I have termed this "*incorporative memory*" (Fuchs 2012). For instance, the submissive behavior of an insecure person, his compliance and anxiousness, belong to a unified pattern of behavior and expression which was acquired in early childhood and now constitutes his personality. Thus, body memory also becomes the carrier of what in sociology has been called the "habitus" (Bourdieu 1990). It may be understood as a set of dispositions, skills, styles, tastes, and ways of acting, which are taken for granted or "go without saying," and which are acquired through the social activities of everyday life. In this way, forms of cultural and class-specific socialization are integrated into the body memory and the manners of a person. "The habitus – embodied history, internalized as a second nature and so forgotten as history – is the active presence of the whole past of which it is the product." (Bourdieu 1990, 56)

We see how the continuous embodiment of existence produces a form of memory which from birth on integrates a person's past into her present bodily constitution. Far from ensuring just an anonymous, pre-reflective existence, the habitual body always forms an excerpt of personal history. It is the expression of our individuality at all levels, not just in the sophisticated ways of self-reflective thought, autobiographical memory, or verbal interaction. This complies with Merleau-Ponty's conception of the continuity of the bodily subject:

> [...] so I am not myself a succession of 'psychic' acts, nor for that matter a nuclear I who brings them together into a synthetic unity, but one single experience inseparable from itself, one single 'living cohesion,' one single temporality which is engaged, from birth, in making itself progressively explicit, and in confirming that cohesion in each successive present. (Merleau-Ponty 1962: 363)

The rational and cognitive understanding of the person binds the conditions for per-sonhood to intentional, conscious acts of remembering. A patient with high-grade dementia would then no longer be a person as he would no longer be able to remember his earlier states of being, perhaps not even his name. However, this understanding of the person separates selfhood from the body. The foundational continuity of a person does not depend on a stock of explicit knowledge and memories or his own biography. It depends, on the one hand, on the subject's bodily self-familiarity: the pre-reflective awareness of self that never fully leaves us. And it is based furthermore on body memory, in other words, on a history accumulated, sedimented in the body and, as such, implicitly always present.

Dementia and Personal Identity

Now we have prepared the ground for a deeper analysis of dementia. How should we conceive and evaluate the identity of demented persons, particularly in later stages of the illness? In what follows, I will develop a phenomenological account of dementia, one which starts from the fundamental loss of reflexivity in dementia patients and then emphasizes the role of body memory for their personal continuity. Finally, I will take a critical look at social constructivist and narrative approaches to the problem of identity in dementia.

Dementia as a Loss of Reflexivity and Meta-Perspective

Since the impairment of short-term memory and temporal orientation belongs to the earliest and most conspicuous symptoms of dementia, it is often regarded as the central disturbance of the disorder. However important this progressive loss of memory may be, the more significant disturbance of dementia only appears in its subsequent course. It is a fundamental impairment of the higher-order capacity for reflexivity and decentering, which was already pointed out by Zutt (1963), Tatossian (1987), and Summa (2014). What is at stake is the particular human capacity for stepping out of one's bodily center and taking a virtual perspective on oneself, which is simultaneously the possible perspective of others—that which Plessner (1928/2019) termed the "eccentric position" of the human being. This crucial function includes a number of interrelated capacities, such as the following:

- *Spatial and temporal orientation.* This is the capacity to rise above the immediacy of current experience in order to locate oneself in an objective geographical and temporal context. This requires mediating one's own bodily orientation in the environment and the moment—in the here and now—with an abstract orientation in objective space and time. Such mediation of two frames of reference becomes particularly manifest in using a map or a calendar.

◆ *Explicit recollection.* Autobiographical memory also requires stepping out of the ongoing current of implicit time (Fuchs 2017b) and the capacity to "re-present" a past experience while being conscious of this stepping out and being able to at least approximately localize the experience within a calendrical time grid. Each dating of events implies stepping out of the immediate stream of time.

◆ *Reflection and self-distancing.* This includes capacities such as reflective thought, taking a stance toward oneself and the situation, anticipation and deliberation of future projects, social perspective-taking, and moral judgment.

◆ *Symbolic or "as-if" function.* This implies the distinction between reality and virtuality, the understanding of metaphors or proverbs, and the capacity of pretending or role-playing, capacities which again require a shifting between two frames of reference (Fuchs 2017c).

Dementia now means, at its core, a disturbance of these reflective and de-centering functions, or to use another term, a loss of meta-perspective. This manifests itself in various phenomena, of which I only mention a selection:

◆ Disturbances of spatial and temporal orientation are a major characteristic of dementia, due to an inability to step out of the here and now. This amounts to an enclosure in the present situation, which can no longer be represented or seen "from above"; hence, maps and calendars become useless. With the loss of overview, the patients' lived space narrows down to the immediate environment, beyond which, already in the imagination, there arises the threat of emptiness, disorientation, and confusion, causing an elementary anxiety.

◆ Explicit recollection is not only impaired because of lost memory contents, but also because the chronological dating of experiences from a superordinate perspective fails, and erratic memories pop up in one's mind without clear localization in time. The loss of meta-perspective and, thus, of a calendrical time grid, leads to a growing fragmentation of the biographical structure of one's life. In later stages of the illness the intentional awareness of remembering itself gets lost. This can result in an unnoticed "shifting" into an earlier phase of life—mistaking one's wife for one's mother, or one's daughter for one's sister, searching for one's childhood home, and so on. Frequently, different phases of one's life overlap or even co-exist simultaneously.

◆ Among the various disturbances of reflexivity and self-distancing I only mention the impairment of perspective-taking (Theory of Mind) and of moral judgment, often leading to disinhibited behavior. This concerns frontotemporal dementia more than Alzheimer's disease, however (Gregory et al. 2002; Lough et al. 2006; Bora et al. 2015). Perseverations and repetitions, which are frequently found in dementia, also indicate an inability to take a distance from a current behavior or situation.

◆ Disturbances of the symbolic or "as-if" function refer to a failure of understanding non-literal language (proverbs, metaphors, irony; cf. Rapp & Wild 2011), but also in a missing distinction of reality and virtuality. Thus, in later stages dementia patients frequently mistake persons in the TV for real people and may try to interact with them. In all these cases, the shifting between two different frames of reference fails, because the required superordinate perspective or "eccentric position" is missing.

If we summarize these disturbances of reflexivity and meta-perspective, we can conceive of dementia as a fundamental disorder of higher-order consciousness, which must also lead to a fragmentation of the continuity of the reflective or narrative self. In this sense, the central disturbance in dementia concerns indeed what Locke considered a person to be, namely

> [. . .] a thinking, intelligent being, that has reason and reflection, and can consider itself as itself, the same thinking thing, in different times and places; which it does only by that consciousness which is inseparable from thinking. (Locke 1997: 302)

This is precisely what patients with dementia are no longer capable of: to reflect on their own existence, to identify certain past activities as "mine," and to anticipate certain future situations as involving "me" (Matthews 2006). What the patients lack, then, is reflective self-consciousness, or the capacity to "consider themselves as themselves." However, as we have seen, the continuity of the person is by no means dependent on reflective or autobiographical continuity; rather, it is fundamentally based on the person's embodied, pre-reflective self. We will now take a closer look at this kind of continuity.

Body Memory in Dementia

If dementia can be properly considered a disturbance of the reflective layers of the self, then the pre-reflective levels become all the more important. The capacity to virtually step out of the situation gets lost, but the patients still experience the world from their bodily center, and the immediate bodily connection to the environment is maintained. To be embodied means to be situated and oriented towards a field of experience as *this* body, as *this* history, *this* point of view (Bullington 2009); and this unique personal orientation conveyed by the lived body still exists in dementia. Hence, the patient will implicitly seek stability in a safe and familiar milieu which provides coherence and shelter against the disruption of reflective orientation in space and time. In contact with others, bodily modes of expression and behavior become more important than cognitive powers and the mostly diminished or fragmented speech acts. The more the patient's behavior may be guided by familiar routines and environmental affordances, the less reflection and meta-perspective is required. This overall shift from abstract orientation, reflection, and symbolic interaction to implicit habits and non-verbal capacities is based on the memory of the body (Fuchs 2012; Summa 2011).

While the progressive loss of explicit (autobiographical and semantic) memory is one of the earliest and most prominent symptoms of Alzheimer's disease, vast ranges of implicit memory remain unimpaired even in late stages of the illness. Accordingly, we can find well retained abilities in all of the previously described forms of body memory. The realization of these abilities is, of course, bound up with appropriate, complementary conditions of the surroundings. Let us look at the different types of body memory in more detail.

1) *Procedural memory.* Recognizing familiar faces and dealing with objects which provide affordances for a certain activity (cutlery, a toothbrush, or such like) remains possible in dementia for a long time, even if the names of persons or objects and their functions can no longer be designated. This corresponds to a dissociation of explicit and implicit memory, which is found in most forms of body memory as a result of the illness. Thus, procedural learning is still possible to a certain extent despite missing recollection; this can be verified by effects of priming or by motor or visual learning tasks (for example maze learning, mirror reading, etc.)—effects which are still comparable to those of healthy elderly people although the patients have no explicit memory of the tasks.[4] Even learning to dance a waltz or the acquisition of other such skills are still possible.[5] Musicians suffering from Alzheimer's disease keep their skills for a long time, often even being able to learn new pieces (Baird et al. 2009).

2) *Situational memory.* As we have seen, body memory conveys our familiarity with situations—surroundings, voices, sounds, and scents with their connotations and atmospheres. This situational memory is also still effective

---

[4] See Rösler et al. (2002), Eldridge et al. (2002), Fleischman et al. (2005), Harrison et al. (2007), and others.

[5] These retained processes of motor learning correspond to the primary cortical localisation of most forms of dementia. Procedural and other forms of body memory are embedded predominantly in subcortical areas of the brain (basal ganglia, cerebellum, amygdala, amongst others) and, for a long period of the illness, remain there unimpaired (Schacter 1992; Squire 2004).

in dementia. Instead of the reflective orientation in space and time, bodily orientation follows the primary directions and relations which the body establishes to the surrounding world, in accordance with the affordances of things: a chair serves "to sit upon," a threshold "to cross," a bed "to rest," and so forth. The bodily habits and dispositions of being in the world can provide patients with elements of security and support. One of the most important tasks in support and care lies, therefore, in the maintenance of an appropriate spatial environment, preferably, of course, their own living space. But care homes can also establish personal spaces which convey at atmosphere of security.

The utmost detailed knowledge of a patient's biography, personal inclinations, and habits allows relatives and careers to bring about continuity and familiarity in the patient's life. Long-known walking routes or locations often have a calming and stabilizing effect, even if the patient no longer has recognizable memories about them at their disposal. Certain sensory stimuli, in particular familiar music, can awake atmospheres, feelings, and even capabilities which are bound to past stages of life, though the memories relating to them have faded away (Sung & Chang 2005). They may also elicit associated autobiographical memories which otherwise escape immediate grasp—as famously described in Proust's experience of the madeleine, the tea-soaked biscuit which evokes the memories of his childhood. Accordingly, body memory may be therapeutically used in manifold ways, for example in art therapy, massage, music, rhythm and dance therapy, animal-based therapy, and so on.[6]

On the other hand, the dissociation of implicit and explicit memory in dementia may also lead to seemingly unmotivated emotions such as sadness, anger, or anxiety, for which the patient cannot name a reason. For example, having experienced a distressing situation, the patient might sometime later, when triggered by a similar object, person or event, become angry or begin to cry—for "no apparent reason" (Sabat 2006). Without an understanding of implicit memory, the person with dementia may then easily be considered as "irrationally hostile," "emotionally labile," or the like. Hence, careful observation and knowledge about the patients' former experiences may help to better understand their reactions.

3) *Incorporative memory.* Body memory also contains the sedimented practices and habits which form a person's character and role identity. Hence,

---

[6] On this, see Filan and Llewellyn-Jones (2006); Guetin et al. (2009); Chancellor et al. (2014); and Karkou & Meekums (2017).

patients with dementia usually show routines and patterns of behavior which correspond to their acquired habitus, though they may no longer fit the current situation. For instance, a patient who formerly worked as a nurse may mistake the care home for her work place, trying to take care of the laundry and giving instructions to other patients. Another patient known for her sense of politeness and hospitality might take great pains to set the table even if no guests are present. For those acquainted with her biography, this characteristic is a part of what makes her the person she is, a surviving fragment of a once much richer identity. Another example may illustrate the effect of formerly incorporated practices:

> A 78-year-old patient in an advanced stage of dementia was mostly incapable of recognizing his surroundings and his relatives any longer. He seemed lethargic, withdrawn, physically frail and was hardly in a position to move about independently any more. One day his two grandchildren visited him and were playing football in front of the house. As a youngster, the patient had played for a long while in a football club; now, he suddenly stood up and played with the boys. In contact with the ball, he appeared as if transformed and much younger; he showed them his skills at dribbling, demonstrated various ball tricks, and gave expert explanations about these. For half an hour, almost nothing was discernible of the illness (case example from my own practice).

The continuity of basal bodily self-experience in dementia is impressively demonstrated in such implicit actualizations of the life story (see also Kontos & Naglie 2009). The once-acquired habitus, such as a professional or sporting activity, is recalled by the relevant situation and its affordances, without requiring a biographical memory or explicit coordination.

4) *Intercorporeal memory.* Admittedly, even the procedural capabilities of body memory are not resistant to the illness in the long run. In the late stages of the process, patients lose not only biographical memories but also (in socalled apraxia) everyday skills, so that even a telephone or a toothbrush can become enigmatic objects. Alongside the sensory-spatial and practical dimensions of body memory, intercorporeality represents the most important source of sustained continuity. The loss of verbal-cognitive powers means that non-verbal, emotional, and bodily communication, as well as the knowhow of everyday modes of behavior, become ever more meaningful. Even in the advanced stages of the illness, the mimetic and gestural expressions of the patient can serve to give a differentiated disclosure of their condition and wishes (Hubbard et al. 2002; Becker et al. 2006; Kruse 2008).

Similarly, sufferers from dementia are particularly sensitive to the affective and atmospheric dimensions of contact. They have the capacity for a diverse range of feelings, display humor, and sometimes surprising quick-wittedness, and, last but not least, have a strong inclination for social bonding. They try to read the state of a relation (acceptance, evaluation, nearness or distance, etc.) from the intonation, facial expression, and gestures of others and react sensitively to social atmospheres, for example to subtle signs of criticism or rejection. The interactions of patients are thereby less determined by conscious reflection or explicit attention to external norms than by the self-evident, pre-reflective nature of their embodied social habitus. Such repertoires of behavior are unjustly discredited as merely "maintaining a facade." Rather, familiar modes of behavior allow the patients to establish affective relations with others and to fall back on basal intercorporeal orientation in situations which are rationally incomprehensible. This is, at the same time, their way of realizing their selves and confirming their existence as a person.

Precisely this need for self-confirmation demonstrates once again how the experience of self is maintained even in advanced dementia. What the patients lose is reflexivity, that higher-level capability of taking a stance toward one's own experience or a momentary situation. Yet the pre-reflective self is not affected by this: indeed, the patient experiences their bodily here-and-now as well as their being-with others above all from an emotional point of view (Summa 2011). This manifests itself, for example, in the shame they feel with regard to failure or incapability, or in the exposure of the body before others; it also shows itself in their feelings of pride or joy in success or appreciation. Last but not least this can be seen in the case of conflicts which arise when the patient is minded to raise borders up around their personal space or to use force to articulate their wishes. The continuity of the basal and thoroughly personally shaped feeling of self should thus prevent us from speaking of a loss of self in dementia.

Relational versus Embodied View of the Person in Dementia

The cognitive and individualistic concept of the self, which we traced back to Descartes and Locke in the second section, has also been criticized from other sides, namely by representatives of social-constructivist or narrativistic views of the person (Kitwood 1997; Sabat & Harré 1992; Radden & Fordyce 2006). For them, personhood is bound up with social relations and the attributions and forms of recognition that result therefrom. The self or the personal identity of demented patients, so argue these authors, is retained in the recognition which others show towards them, and in the narrative projections of the patient's identity which others provide in their place. Thus, Kitwood defines the notion of the person as "the standing or status that is bestowed upon one human being by others, in the context of relationship and social being" (Kitwood 1997: 8), and concludes:

> In dementia many aspects of the psyche that had, for a long time, been individual and "internal," are again made over to the interpersonal milieu. Memory may have faded, but something of the past is known; identity remains intact, because others hold it in place; thoughts may have disappeared, but there are still interpersonal processes. (Kitwood 1997: 69)

On the basis of a narrative concept of identity, Radden and Fordyce take a similar position:

> The very self-awareness required to possess an identity depends upon and grows out of the contribution, and particularly the recognition, of other persons. (Radden & Fordyce 2006: 72)

Finally, arguing for a social constructivist view of the self, Sabat and Harrè regard the Alzheimer disease sufferer as a "semiotic subject":

> Personhood can be an interpersonal discursive construction, a property of conversations […] The mind is no more than, but no less than, a privatized part of the "general conversation." (Sabat & Harré 1994: 145 f.)

The view that the self is mainly articulated through language and social relations has also determined the majority of studies on evidence of the persistence of self in dementia: they have usually focused on discourse, language, and narrative (Saunders 1998; Sabat 2002; Beard 2004; Addis & Tippett 2004; Surr 2006; Fazio & Mitchell 2009), whereas only one study has investigated embodied selfhood in dementia (Kontos 2003, 2004; see Cadell & Clare 2010 for an overview).

Yet, as meaningful as intersubjectivity for the concept of person is, without a foundation in the subjectivity of the patient themselves, such attributions, narrative substitutes, or representations of interest by proxy are without adequate basis. Clearly, these have their significance for person-centered care, but they are first borne and supported by the modes of expression and behavior in which the personal identity and selfhood of the patient manifests itself right up to the end. Hence, even granted that the personal self is also relational in nature, such relations are always directed towards others as embodied subjects, and not as mere intersections of relations or projection surfaces.

Founding the self in dementia on an externalist or discursive account misses the first-person perspective or the patient's primary self-awareness in favor of a problematic social constructivist model of the self. As we have seen, an embodied view of dementia also emphasizes the implicit relations which the lived body establishes to the environment, and the ecological niche which conveys a sense of familiarity and belonging to the patient. However, it regards body memory, intercorporeality, and inter-affectivity as the basis of any person-centered approach to dementia, particularly in later phases of the illness. By contrast, narrative and constructivist views run the risk of "constructing" the patient instead of carefully perceiving his or her maintained personality in his or her bodily expressions and behavior. Moreover, they reach their limits when the patient's capacity for verbal interaction subsides, whereas the embodied self is still attainable and tangible even in the last stages of dementia.

An embodied concept of the person rests on a double foundation: on the one hand, on the continuity of organic life, which the body establishes even through phases of unconsciousness; on the other hand, on bodily subjectivity, which maintains a continuity of selfhood through body memory even when the capacity for self-knowledge has been lost (Fuchs 2017b). The persistence of the person is therefore valid both from a third-person point of view, related to the organic body (*Körper*), and from the experience of the first person, related to the lived body (*Leib*). Personal existence means primarily bodily selfhood and being alive, from the beginning to the end. Reflective self-awareness, rationality, and autonomy are, to give an analogy, like the fruit on a tree, namely the appearance and product of an entire life, and cannot be separated from its bearer. They are abilities that are always actualized only for certain periods of time, but which are not sufficient to ensure the continuity of the person as such. Moreover, making them the sole condition for the attribution of personal status, as Peter Singer and other ethicists advocate, excludes a wide circle of people from being persons: newborns, severely retarded people, and people with advanced dementia.

This is not intended to deny the importance of autobiographically and narratively conveyed identity. Amnesia and dementia diseases show unequivocally that the loss of explicit memory and autobiographical knowledge also fundamentally question one's own selfhood. Conversely, however, self-reflection, memory, and narration must also be embedded in basal bodily self-acquaintance in order to constitute personal identity. In this respect, implicit and explicit, bodily and autobiographical memory contribute equally to personal identity. The loss of higher cognitive and self-reflective abilities such as self-knowledge or autonomous decision-making undoubtedly means a massive impairment of characteristics that we attribute to a healthy, adult person. All the more important, though, are the interpersonal and relational forms of personhood and recognition that are able to replace those lost abilities to a certain extent. But this does not mean that the concept of person dissolves into mere relationality: all interpersonal relationships remain bound to the bodily appearance and continuity of the person.

Conclusion

The concept of embodied personhood and history is able to change our image of dementia. In place of a brain- and cognition-centered perspective, we may adopt the view of the patients in their own individual embodiment, which, for its part, is embedded in social and environmental contexts. Even when dementia robs patients of their explicit memories, they still retain their body memory, that means, their familiarity with environments, habits, sensory and motor memories. And, instead of relying merely on rationality and autonomy, their self can be seen as being primarily based on intercorporeality and inter-affectivity, which remain in place despite the progress of the illness.

There is no question that higher-order capacities such as reflective thought and autobiographical memory are crucial for our everyday sense of identity—our knowing the person that we are. In that sense, people with severe dementia have undeniably lost part of their identity as persons. However, the memory of the body compromises a different, submerged history of the self. Its temporality does not follow the linear progress of the autobiographical life story, from which we can purposefully retrieve memories. In body memory, the past persists more as an organically accumulated and sedimented history, and it becomes effective in our personal forms of perception, behavior, and interaction, without our being conscious of their particular origins. It is on this continuity and memory of the lived body that the identity of the patient remains founded.

Without doubt, the capacities and habits mediated by the body are part of the patients' individual history, even though the patient may not be able to re-member having learnt those capacities. Contrary to Locke's view, our identity reaches further back than our explicit recollection. In our habitus, in our bodily being, we manifest ourselves as persons no less than in our cognitive and re-flective powers. If we understand selfhood as primarily bodily, we therefore ar-rive at a different perception of the patient with dementia: no longer as a person whom rationality and personality have abandoned, but rather as a person whose personhood can be precisely realized as both bodily and intercorporeal, so long as they can continue to live in the appropriate spatial, atmospheric, and social surroundings.

A concept of person grounded solely in rationality and reflection inevitably stigmatizes people with severe cognitive deficits. By contrast, bringing in a concept of person orientated towards embodiment and intercorporeality, the response and relational capabilities of patients become a significant founda-tion of their personhood—such as the ability to give expression to joy, grate-fulness, sorrow, or fear that is still preserved. This elementary intercorporeal expressivity and responsiveness is the basis of the claim for respect, recognition and dignity which persons suffering from dementia also raise towards others. Their individuality remains present in familiar sights, smells, and melodies, in their dealing with things and their familiarity with other people—even though they are no longer able to account for the origin of this familiarity, nor to tell their life story. This is because the fundamental continuity of the person exists in the unified connection of their life, in the uninterrupted temporality of their body.

References

Addis, D. R., L. J. Tippett. 2004. "Memory of myself: Autobiographical memory and identity in Alzheimer's disease." *Memory* 12: 56–74.

Bachelard, G. 1964. *The Poetics of Space*. D. Russell (trans.) Boston: Beacon. (Originally published 1958.)

Baird, A., S. Samson. 2009. "Memory for music in Alzheimer's disease: Unforgettable?" *Neuropsychology Review* 19: 85–101.

Beard, R. L. 2004. "In their voices: Identity preservation and experiences of Alzheimer's disease." *Journal of Aging Studies* 18: 415–428.

Becker, S., R. Kaspar, A. Kruse. 2006. "Die Bedeutung unterschiedlicher Referenzgruppen für die Beurteilung der Lebensqualität demenzkranker Menschen." *Zeitschrift für Gerontologie und Geriatrie* 39: 350–357.

Bergson, H. 1988. *Matter and Memory*. Nancy Margaret Paul and W. Scott Palmer (trans.) Cambridge MA & London: Zone Books.

Biran, M. de 1953. *Influence de l'habitude sur la faculté de penser*. Paris: PUF.

Bora, E., Walterfang, M., Velakoulis, D. 2015. "Theory of mind in behavioral-variant frontotemporal dementia and Alzheimer's disease: A meta-analysis." *Journal of Neurology, Neurosurgery & Psychiatry* 86: 714–719.

Bourdieu, P. 1990. *The Logic of Practice*. Cambridge: Cambridge University Press.

Bullington, J. 2009. "Being body: The dignity of human embodiment." In Nordenfelt, L. (ed.) *Dignity in Care for Older People*. Hoboken/NJ: John Wiley & Sons (pp. 54–76).

Butler, J. 1736/1877. "Of personal identity." In J. Angus (ed.) *The Analogy of Religion*. London: Allman & Sawers (pp. 211–215).

Caddell, L. S., L. Clare. 2010. "The impact of dementia on self and identity: A systematic review." *Clinical Psychology Review* 30: 113–126.

Casey, E. S. 1984. "Habitual body and memory in Merleau-Ponty." *Man and World*, 17: 279–297.

Eldridge, L. L., D. Masterman, B. J. Knowlton. 2002. "Intact implicit habit learning in Alzheimer's disease." *Behavioral Neuroscience* 116: 722–726.

Fazio, S., D. B. Mitchell. 2009. "Persistence of self in individuals with Alzheimer's disease: Evidence from language and visual recognition." *Dementia* 8: 39–59.

Filan, S. L., R. H. Llewellyn-Jones. 2006. "Animal-assisted therapy for dementia: A review of the literature." *International Psychogeriatrics* 18: 597–611.

Fleischman, D. A., R. Wilson, J. D. Gabriele, J. Schneider, J. Bienias, D. A. Bennett. 2005. "Implicit memory and Alzheimer's disease neuropathology." *Brain* 128: 2006–2015.

Fuchs, T. 2012. "The phenomenology of body memory." In *Body Memory, Metaphor and Movement*. Koch, S., Fuchs, T., Summa, M., Müller, C. (eds.) Amsterdam: John Benjamins, (pp. 9–22).

Fuchs, T. 2017a. "Intercorporeality and interaffectivity." In C. Meyer, J. Streeck, S. Jordan (eds.) *Intercorporeality: Emerging Socialities in Interaction*. Oxford: Oxford University Press (pp. 3–24).

Fuchs, T. 2017b. "Self across time: The diachronic unity of bodily existence." *Phenomenology and the Cognitive Sciences* 16: 291–315.

Fuchs, T. 2017c. "The 'as if' function and its loss in schizophrenia." In Summa, M., Fuchs, T., Vanzago, L. (eds.) *Imagination and Social Perspectives: Approaches from Phenomenology and Psychopathology*. New York, London: Routledge (pp. 83–98).

Fuchs, T. 2018. *Ecology of the Brain: The Phenomenology and Biology of the Embodied Mind*. Oxford: Oxford University Press.

Garrett, B. 1998. *Personal Identity and Self-Consciousness*. London: Routledge.

Gibson, J. 1979. *The Ecological Approach to Visual Perception*. Boston: Houghton Mifflin.

Golby, A., G. Silverbergt, E. Race, S. Gabrieli, J. O'Shea, K. Knierim, G., Stebbins, J. Gabrieli. 2005. "Memory encoding in Alzheimer's disease: An fMRI study of explicit and implicit memory." *Brain* 128: 773–787.

Gregory, C., S. Lough, V. Stone, S. Erzinclioglu, L. Martin, S. Baron-Cohen, J. R. Hodges. 2002. "Theory of mind in patients with frontal variant frontotemporal dementia and Alzheimer's disease: Theoretical and practical implications." *Brain* 125: 752–764.

Guetin, S., F. Portet, M. C. Picot, C. Pommié, M. Messaoudi, L. Djabelkir, A. L Olsen, M. M., Cano, E. Lecourt, J. Touchon. 2009. "Effect of music therapy on anxiety and depression in patients with Alzheimer's-type dementia: Randomised, controlled study." *Dementia and Geriatric Cognitive Disorders* 28: 36–46.

Harrison, B. E., G. Son, J. Kim, A. L. Whall. 2007. "Preserved implicit memory in dementia: A potential model of care." *American Journal of Alzheimer's Disease & Other Dementias* 22: 286–293.

Hubbard, G., Cook, A., Tester, S., Downs, M. 2002. "Beyond words: Older people with dementia using and interpreting nonverbal behavior." *Journal of Aging Studies* 16: 155–167.

Husserl, E. 1991. *On the Phenomenology of the Consciousness of Internal Time*. John Barnett Brough (trans.) Dordrecht: Kluwer.

Karkou, V., B. Meekums. 2017. "Dance movement therapy for dementia." *Cochrane Database of Systematic Reviews* (2).

Kitwood, T. 1997. *Dementia Reconsidered: The Person comes First*. Buckingham, UK: Open University Press.

Klein, S. 2013. "The sense of diachronic personal identity." *Phenomenology and the Cognitive Sciences* 12, 791–811.

Kontos, P. 2003. "'The Painterly hand': Embodied consciousness and Alzheimer's disease." *Journal of Aging Studies* 17: 151–170.

Kontos, P. C. 2004. "Ethnographic reflections on selfhood, embodiment and Alzheimer's disease." *Ageing & Society* 24: 829–849.

Kontos, P. C., G. Naglie. 2009. "Tacit knowledge of caring and embodied selfhood." *Sociology of Health and Illness* 31: 688–704.

Kruse, A. 2008. "Der Umgang mit demenzkranken Menschen als ethische Aufgabe." *Archiv für Wissenschaft und Praxis der sozialen Arbeit* 39: 14–21.

Locke, J. 1997. *An Essay Concerning Human Understanding*. London: Penguin.

Lough, S., C. M. Kipps, C. Treise, P. Watson, J. R. Blair, J. R. Hodges. 2006. "Social reasoning, emotion and empathy in frontotemporal dementia." *Neuropsychologia* 44: 950–958.

Matthews, E. 2006. "Dementia and the identity of the person." In Hughes, J. C., Louw, S. J., Sabat, S. R. (eds.) *Dementia: Mind, Meaning, and the Person*. Oxford: Oxford University Press (pp. 163–177).

Maurer, K., Volk, S., Gerbaldo, H. 1997. "Auguste D and Alzheimer's Disease." *The Lancet* 349(9064): 1546–1549.

McMahan, J. 2003. *The Ethics of Killing: Problems at the Margins of Life*. Oxford: Oxford University Press.

Merleau-Ponty, M. 1962. *Phenomenology of Perception*. Colin Smith (trans.) London: Routledge & Kegan Paul.

Parfit, D. 1984. *Reasons and Persons*. Oxford: Clarendon Press.

Plessner, H. 2019. *Levels of Organic life and the Human: An Introduction to Philosophical Anthropology*. New York: Fordham University Press. (German original published 1928.)

Radden, J., J. M. Fordyce. 2006. "Into the darkness: Losing identity with dementia." In J. C. Hughes, S. J. Louw, S. R Rabat (eds.) *Dementia: Mind, Meaning, and the Person*. Oxford: Oxford University Press (pp. 71–87).

Rapp, A. M., B. Wild. 2011. "Nonliteral language in Alzheimer dementia: A review." *Journal of the International Neuropsychological Society* 17: 207–218.

Rösler, A., E. Seifritz, K. Kräuchi, D. Spoerl, I. Brokuslaus, S. M. Proserpi, A. Gendre, E. Savaskan, M. Hofmann. 2002. "Skill learning in patients with moderate Alzheimer's disease: A prospective pilot-study of waltz-lessons." *International Journal of Geriatric Psychiatry* 17: 1155–1156.

Sabat, S. R. 2002. "Surviving manifestations of selfhood in Alzheimer's disease: A case study." *Dementia* 1: 25–36.

Sabat, S. R. 2006. "Implicit memory and people with Alzheimer's disease. Implication for caregiving." *American Journal of Alzheimer's Disease and other Dementias* 21: 11–14

Sabat, S. R., R. Harré. 1992. "The construction and deconstruction of self in Alzheimer's disease." *Ageing and Society* 12: 443–461.

Sabat, S. R., R. Harré. 1994. "The Alzheimer's disease sufferer as a semiotic subject." *Philosophy, Psychiatry, & Psychology* 1: 145–160.

Saunders, P. A. 1998. "'My brain's on strike'—the construction of identity through memory accounts by dementia patients." *Research on Aging* 20: 65–90.

Schacter, D. L. 1987. "Implicit memory: History and current status." *Journal of Experimental Psychology: Learning, Memory and Cognition* 13: 501–518.

Schacter, D. L. 1992. "Understanding implicit memory: A cognitive neuroscience approach." *American Psychologist* 47: 559–569.

Schacter, D. L. 1996. *Searching for Memory: The Brain, the Mind, and the Past*. New York: Basic Books.

Shoemaker, S. 1970. "Persons and their pasts." *American Philosophical Quarterly* 7: 269–285

Singer, P. 1979. *Practical Ethics*. Cambridge: Cambridge University Press.

Squire, L. R. 2004. "Memory systems of the Brain: A brief history and current perspective." *Neurobiology of Learning and Memory* 82: 171–177.

Stern, D. N. 1985. *The Interpersonal World of the Infant: A View from Psychoanalysis and Developmental Psychology*. New York: Basic Books.

Stern, D. N. 1998. "The process of therapeutic change involving implicit knowledge: Some implications of developmental observations for adult psychotherapy." *Infant Mental Health Journal* 19: 300–308.

Summa, M. 2011. "Das Leibgedächtnis: Ein Beitrag aus der Phänomenologie Husserls." *Husserl Studies* 27: 173–196.

Summa, M. 2014. "The disoriented self: Layers and dynamics of self-experience in dementia and schizophrenia." *Phenomenology and the Cognitive Sciences* 13: 477–496.

Sung, H., A. M. Chang. 2005. "Use of preferred music to decrease agitated behaviors in older people with dementia: A review of the literature." *Journal of Clinical Nursing* 14: 1133–1140.

Surr, C. A. 2006. "Preservation of self in people with dementia living in residential care: A socio-biographical approach." *Social Science and Medicine* 62: 1720–1730.

Tatossian, A. 1987. "Phénoménologie des états démentiels." *Psychologie Médicale* 19: 1205–1207.

Trevarthen, C. (1993). "The self born in intersubjectivity." In U. Neisser (ed.) *The Perceived Self: Ecological and Interpersonal Sources of Self-knowledge*. Cambridge: Cambridge University Press (pp. 121–173).

Zahavi, D. 1999. *Self-awareness and Alterity: A Phenomenological Investigation*. Evanstone: Northwestern University Press.

Zahavi, D. 2006. *Subjectivity and Selfhood: Investigating the First-Person Perspective*. Cambridge, MA: MIT Press.

Zutt, J. 1963. *Auf dem Wege zu einer aAnthropologischen Psychiatrie: Gesammelte Aufsätze*. Berlin Heidelberg: Springer.

Chapter 10

The Cyclical Time of the Body and the Linear Time of Modernity

Introduction

The conception of time as a linear, uniform, and continually progressing process appears to us today as so self-evident that we easily forget that it is a concept that was developed only with European modernity. Concepts of time in earlier cultures were based primarily on the cyclical recurrence of cosmic and earthly processes. Rhythms of day and night, seasons, ebb and flow, lunar and planetary cycles determined social processes and were carried over into cultic practices. Myth and rite know no real progress into the future; rather, rituals reenact a mythical past in which the community participates in a mimetic form, so that the originary moment can be renewed again and again (Levy-Bruhl 1966; Eliade 1959). Society's chronological order is therefore not yet emancipated from natural processes. Frequently, early cultures lack an abstract concept of time as detached from rhythmic processes or actions altogether. This applies in particular to hunter-gatherer societies, namely before the organization of agriculture created the need for time measurement and calendars (Elias 2007: 33–34, 40–43).

A linearly directed conception of time developed first in Judaism and Christianity with the idea of a history of salvation as a process directed into the future. This process reaches its goal in the appearance of the messiah or in the Parousia of the Lord: then, indeed, time itself will end again (Achtner et al. 1998). However, the linear conception of time finds its actual shape in the scientific-technological advances of modernity: human cultural products, from the mechanical clock in the fourteenth century to the continually accelerated means of transportation in the nineteenth and twentieth centuries, create and establish the idea of time as a continually progressive flow in close connection with Newtonian physics (Elias 2007). Here, time was conceived as a homogeneous, steadily quantifiable arrow. On this arrow, each event can only hold one irreversibly transient position; for time itself runs on and does not return. But, this linear, homogeneous time, abstracted from all concrete processes, does not show itself in the natural world pregiven to humans—here we encounter

In Defense of the Human Being. Thomas Fuchs, Oxford University Press. © Suhrkamp Verlag 2021.
DOI: 10.1093/oso/9780192898197.003.0011

initially only cyclical, recurring, or finalizing processes. Rather, the linear concept of time was first constructed in the cultural world shaped by humans and then transferred to the cosmic sphere.

However, cyclical time is not simply overcome. This is because it denotes not only a particular level of culture, but rather the temporal form of the processes of life themselves, and closely connected to this, the temporality of the *lived body*. From the periodic nature of physiological processes, such as heartbeat, respiration, circadian rhythms, or hormonal cycles, to the recurrent, automatic actions and habits of the body, all life lived in a pre-reflexive way is shaped by a cyclical structure. This structure, indeed, founds and carries all projects which are linearly directed towards the future. However, the connection between cyclical and linear time, in both the individual enactment of life as well as in social processes, by no means proceeds only harmoniously, but also frequently antagonistically. If cyclical processes are neglected, this can, as we will see, lead to physical or psychological as well as to social disorders.

In the following I will represent the cyclical time of the body in its most important aspects in order to then examine its relationship to the linear time of the societal processes of modernity. A concluding glance will be given to some psychopathological phenomena, which can be described as the result of a conflict between the cyclical and linear order of time.

The Processes of Life and their Cyclical Time

The temporality of a living organism is characterized in principle by periodically recalled processes. Life constitutes and reproduces itself in contradistinction to the permanent processes of decay, to the entropy of inorganic nature. It establishes an inner-outer distinction which nevertheless remains precarious, that is, its conservation depends on metabolic exchange with the environment (Jonas 1966). While with plants, fixed as they are in place, this exchange proceeds continuously, animal organisms are detached from spatial localization and confront the environment through their senses and autonomous movements. But here the periods become the form in which organisms maintain their internal order: recurrent deficiencies must be balanced by counter-regulation, substance-seeking, and intake. Metabolism and homeostatic regulation do not take place statically or continuously, but rather do so in the constant change of ingestion and excretion, expenditure and regeneration, waking and sleeping, "ergotropic," and "trophotropic," phases.

Physiological processes are marked, therefore, by various cycles which are coordinated with each other and which are simultaneously synchronized with cosmic rhythms: such as the daily rhythm of hormone secretion, wake-sleep cycles, and energy balance (measurable as the circadian rise and fall of body temperature), the high and low points of activity in the course of a day or year, and so forth.[1] Moreover, instinctual impulses are also cyclically recurring. These are impulses in which the animal becomes aware of a certain deficiency, such as in thirst, hunger, the motor or the sex drive.

With this instinctual direction, the felt "not yet" of possible fulfilment awakens as well (Jonas 1966: 99 ff.). In this directionality of anticipated satisfaction lies a central root of the experience of time. Deficiency and need open up a differential of time, or a "timespan," which is primarily experienced as an appetitive tension—of course only up until the achieved satisfaction. The specifically object-orientated arcs of suspense are formed by the *affects*, which bridge the delay of satisfaction in experience and accompany the movement toward the desired object. In order that the target remains at the center of attention during the approach, it must be emotionally invested. Hunting is motivated by desire and aggression, flight, conversely, by avoidance and fear. With the conclusion of the respective arcs of tension, that is, with satisfaction, a new phase sets in with a correspondingly changed mood, such as languor or relaxation, until a new directionality emerges. This cyclical dynamic of lack, urge, expectation, desire, lust, and fulfilment is both the subjective side and the motivating force of the processes of self-preservation which constitute animal life. They lay the basis for the corresponding cyclical temporal experience, without already bringing about an overarching linear time perspective.

Yet also, in the micro-temporality of experience, periodical bodily processes play a formative, if not a constitutive, role. Thus, respiratory movement and heartbeat produce a constant underlying rhythmization of the stream of consciousness, even if this is for the most part not consciously recognized. On a neurobiological level, recent research suggests that the central integration of such rhythmic bodily signals forms the basis of our sense of the duration of time. This integration is bound to several brain regions such as the insular and the inferior parietal cortex, the middle temporal gyrus, and the operculum (Craig 2009; Wittmann 2009, 2011). Thus, the interoceptive experience of one's own body not only provides a pre-reflective self-awareness, but also underlies the diachronic continuity of the embodied self (Fuchs 2017). Yet the sense of temporal continuity does not seem to be dependent on external sense perception. In experiments with complete exteroceptive sensory deprivation in an

---

[1] These endogenous rhythms have their neurobiological basis mostly in the hypothalamus (in particular, the *nucleus suprachiasmaticus* for rhythmic motor activity, food and liquid intake, or sleep-wake cycle; and the *nucleus ventromedialis* for temperature levels and food intake, glucose and insulin levels, and others).

isolation tank, subjects usually experience feelings of time extension or time-lessness; nevertheless, the basic sense of temporal continuity remains intact, obviously because the constancy of internal bodily experience is not suspended (Baxton et al. 1954; Lilly 1977; Kjellgren et al. 2008).

Moreover, according to experimental studies, the precision of the estimation of time also depends on the individual capability of interoception, especially on the capacity for perceiving rhythmic bodily signals (Meissner & Wittmann 2011; Pollatos et al. 2014). Similarly, the subjective experience of the dur-ation of time varies depending on the motivation, arousal, or relaxation of the body, which is manifested in heart and breathing rates, amongst other things (Wittmann 2009). Sympathicotonic arousal and parasympathicotonic relax-ation come with different experiences of time—think about the sense of time when positively aroused as opposed to one of tiredness or boredom. Above all, the vital increase of drive in manic states as well as the inhibition of drive in de-pression lead to changes in the experience of time, namely to a felt acceleration in one case and to a stretching of time in the other (Fuchs 2001, 2013; Bschor et al. 2004).

Finally, the subjective experience of *presence* in no way forms a linear con-tinuum either. The present moment is not a mathematical point on a timeline; rather, it is extended in the form of intervals, in which events are rhythmically combined into meaningful groups (Kiverstein 2010). Various findings point to an interval duration of the experienced present of approximately 3 seconds (see Pöppel 1997, 2000: 63 ff.).[2] This is noticeable in the spontaneous segmentation that occurs when one listens to the regular ticking of a metronome. Through ac-centuation, beats of twos or threes emerge in our minds (1-2, 1-2, etc.; or 1-2-3, 1-2-3, etc.). However, this grouping only works up to an interval of 2 to 3 seconds between the beats; beyond that only single beats can be heard, and grouping is no longer possible (Szelag et al. 1996; London 2002). Similarly, the perspectival perception of ambiguous or bi-stable figures, such as Necker's Cube, or the ge-stalt perception of Rubin's Vase (is it a vase or two faces?), switches around every 3 seconds spontaneously (Kornmeier et al. 2007). Lastly, spontaneous speech is also rhythmically structured, so that the average duration of a verse line is about 3 seconds (Pöppel 2000: 85 f.). In their interactions with one another, mothers and babies already show regular turn-taking in vocalization or other

---

[2] There are also other time windows of subjective experience, e.g., for the integration of stimuli into one simultaneous sensory experience (ranging from tens to a few hundreds of milliseconds, depending on the sense modality), or the longer time window of working memory (up to 100 seconds) (see Wittmann 2011). Here I restrict the account to the sense of subjective presence.

expressive gestures at a pace of 2–3 seconds and thereby build a shared present (Malloch 1999). The rhythmic or musical nature of early intercorporeality is also highlighted by Stern's concept of "vitality affects," meaning the intensity contours of mutual bodily expressions such as surging, bursting, accelerating, slowing-down, fading away, etc., which are mostly bound to a time frame of a few seconds (Stern, 2004, 2010).

To sum up, action and perception are integrated into respective meaningful units within extended temporal windows that lend a "width" to the present, though obviously these windows or intervals are somehow connected.[3] In other words, the experienced present as belonging together, or the "extended now"— described famously by Husserl (1991) as the unity of *primary impression, retention*, and *protention*—tends towards intervals of a few seconds' duration.

All of these findings prove that the temporality of implicit, bodily experience is not experienced in a linear way but rather rhythmically or cyclically, as long as this pre-reflexive experience is not overlaid by an explicit reference to the anticipated future or the remembered past. It is only this reference which produces an overarching and mostly linear perspective of time. Kant famously conceptualized time as a form of the "... inner sense, i.e., of the intuition of our self and our inner state" (Kant 1998: B49), which, however, remained an abstract and formal definition. This transcendental form of time can indeed be understood phenomenologically as an "inner," that is to say *bodily* sense of time. It was William James who already doubted Kant's pure and disembodied transcendental apperception:

> I am as confident as I am of anything that, in myself, the stream of thinking (which I recognize emphatically as a phenomenon) is only a careless name for what, when scrutinized, reveals itself to consist chiefly of the stream of my breathing. The "I think" which Kant said must be able to accompany all my objects, is the "I breathe" which actually does accompany them. (James 1904: 491)

Of course, holding one's breath does not interrupt the stream of consciousness; stating this James is undoubtedly going too far. Still the breath is, as we have seen, just another form of the rhythmization of consciousness through varied periodical and cyclic bodily processes. Understanding consciousness as entirely embodied enables us to state the following thesis: *the primary and implicit form of time experience reveals the rhythmic-dynamic structure of the lived body and of the processes of life which underlie this very experience.* Hence, if Merleau-Ponty's claim is justified that "we must understand time as the subject, and the subject

---

[3] The question of how this connection is achieved through overlap or higher level units has been considered for example by Dainton (2010) and Wittmann (2011), but cannot be discussed here in more detail.

as time" (Merleau-Ponty 1962: 376), in other words, if temporality in this way constitutes the subject, this must be brought together with its embodiment: "I am my body [...] and yet at the same time my body is as it were a 'natural' subject, a provisional sketch of my total being" (ibid. 178). This way, the cyclical time of life and the body can be understood as the "sketch," or the basic form, of experience in its temporal structure.

The Cyclical Structure of Body Memory

Until now, I have considered the temporality of the body with regard to the recurrent cycles of desire and satisfaction, and the micro-periods of the bodily present. I move now to another cyclical temporal structure, which manifests itself in *habituality*, or the structure of habit, and which I have already described as implicit or *body memory* in Chapter 9. This memory is, at base, radically different from explicit, autobiographical memory, or remembering: while the latter shows a linear form of time, that is to say the experiences line up in an arrow of time directed into the past and are so remembered, body memory by contrast consists in repetition, the "re-enactment" of the experienced, the learned, or habitualized, without the past being remembered as such (Fuchs 2012).

I have already pointed out that the distinction between the two kinds of memory goes back to Maine de Biran and Henri Bergson, the latter of whom speaks of a *souvenir-image* and a *mémoire-habitude* (Bergson 1988; Summa 2011). The *souvenir-image* or image memory registers the events of the past successively and reproduces them as episodes in memory; the *mémoire-habitude* or habitual memory, on the contrary, does not *represent* the past but rather *reenacts* it implicitly or unconsciously in bodily-practical implementations. In such a way, a poem learned by heart through repetition detaches from the biographical past and becomes part of the present sensorimotor or bodily disposition:

> And, in fact, the lesson once learned bears upon it no mark which betrays its origin and classes it in the past; it is part of my present, exactly like my habit of walking or of writing; it is lived and acted, rather than represented. (Bergson 1988: 79)

Repetition and practice are the primary ways in which habits of movement, perception, and behavior anchor themselves in body memory, starting with walking upright, through learning to read and write to the use of instruments such as playing the violin, or typing with a keyboard. Bodily learning consists mainly in the gradual *forgetting* of what initially had to be taught or shown explicitly: learned action becomes a part of implicit bodily memory—becomes part of our "flesh and blood." From repetition results *automatization*, a process that integrates single movements within a uniform temporal gestalt, which is incorporated into unreflective bodily enactments (Fuchs 2012). One then no longer knows how one does what one self-evidently does—such as driving a car or dancing a waltz. The *knowing how* lies in the limbs and senses of the body, on which we come to rely. This melting of repeated experiences into body memory can also be described as *implication*. It is particularly favored by rhythmic repetition, be it in melodies, meter, or rhyming, or be it in the rhythms and temporal forms of movement, such as walking, dancing, or skiing.

Thus, here we once again meet the rhythmic-periodical structure of immediate bodily enactment. Yet, this structure is now integrated within an overarching cyclical structure through body memory, namely in the habit or habituality of the body. It conveys our underlying experience of familiarity with the world, and our experience of sameness and recurrence in the change of situations. Primarily formed in early childhood, habituality modifies and alters itself in the course of life—body memory displays a lifelong if waning plasticity. Nevertheless, the temporality of existence remains bound to a basic cyclical structure—it is also repetition in every moment, the recurrence of the familiar and the similar. The surprising and the new can only emerge against this given background.

Notably, the cyclical character of body memory shows itself in situations in which it generates not only a familiarity but also a literal re-experience of past events. That is the case, for example, if I return to a childhood place after many years, and suddenly *my seeing from back then* repeats itself, indeed, my whole bodily condition is reawakened as in a *déjà-vu* or *déjà-vecu*-experience. While explicit memory normally makes the past present in a merely representative way, i.e., in its objective distance from the present, in *déjà-vecu* experiences the past and the present literally seem to coincide. This corresponds to Proust's term "*mémoire involontaire*," best known from the first volume of *À la recherche du temps perdu* in the recognition of the "Madeleine," a tea-soaked cake, the taste of which opens the door to a forgotten past:

> No sooner had the warm liquid mixed with the crumbs touched my palate than a shiver ran through me and I stopped, intent upon the extraordinary thing that was happening to me. An exquisite pleasure had invaded my senses, something isolated, detached, with no suggestion of its origin. (Proust 1992: 60)

This feeling of happiness results from the union of present and past, namely from the awakening of "this old, dead moment which the magnetism of an identical moment has travelled so far to importune, to disturb, to raise up out of the very depths of my being" (Proust 1992: 63). Implicitly contained in the present sensory impression, the past now unfolds itself out of the body memory to form Marcel's explicit remembering of his childhood in Combray.[4] In the final volume of the *Recherche*, Proust describes this recurrence as an extra-temporal (one could also say, cyclical-present) experience, which is even able to overcome the linear temporality of *being-towards-death*:

> This explained why it was that my anxiety on the subject of my death had ceased at the moment when I had unconsciously recognized the taste of the little Madeleine, since the being which at that moment I had been was an extra-temporal being and therefore unalarmed by the vicissitudes of the future. This being had only come to me, only manifested itself outside of activity an immediate enjoyment, on those rare occasions when the miracle of an analogy had made me escape from the present. And only this being had the power to perform that task which had always defeated the efforts of my memory and my intellect, the power to make me rediscover days that were long past, the Time that was Lost. (Proust 1993: 223)

Beneath both a passing lifetime and those memories lined up in a linear way in autobiographical memory one can find a layer of bodily experience that is not organized sequentially, nor that simply passes by, but rather constantly grows through new experiences. This layer is also able to produce "subterranean connections," as it were, between distant points of time in biography.

Now, it is by no means solely positive experience which enters body memory in this way. Traumatic experiences can also inscribe themselves into body memory and later, through similar situations, awaken once more, often in the form of an intensive present recurrence, as if the trauma were happening once again (so-called "flashback memories"). A striking example of traumatic body memory can be found in the autobiography of the Jewish writer Aharon Appelfeld, who had to stay hidden in the forests of Ukraine as a boy during the Second World War:

> More than fifty years have passed since the end of the war. I have forgotten much, even things that were very close to me – places in particular, dates, and the names of people – and yet I can still sense those days in every part of my body. Whenever it rains, it's cold, or a fierce wind is blowing, I am taken back to the ghetto, to the camp, or to the forests where I spent many days. Memory, it seems, has deep roots in the body." – "The cells of my body apparently remember more than my mind which is supposed to remember. For years after the war, I would walk neither in the middle

---

[4] One thinks of the principle of association; however, as Bergson has shown, this atomistic conception decomposes the original unity of bodily awareness, the components of which are not combined but are rather *implied* in an overall primary experience. It is precisely this holistic experience that is awakened in body memory and which is only then explicated in individual components: "I smell a rose and immediately confused recollections of childhood come back to my memory. In truth these recollections have not been called up by the perfume of the rose: *I breathe them in with the very scent; it means all that to me*" (Bergson 1910: 161; italics mine).

of the sidewalk nor in the middle of the road. I always clung to the walls, always staying in the shade, and always walking rapidly, as if I were slipping away. [...] Sometimes, just the aroma of a certain dish, or the dampness of shoes or a sudden noise is enough to take me back in the middle of the war [...] The war has infiltrated my bones." (Appelfeld 2009: 50, 90)

Here it is not a single traumatic event, so much as a whole phase of life which has left its traces behind in body memory, and these traces are deeper and more durable than autobiographical memories: certain body sensations, perceptions of touch, odor, or hearing, indeed even weather conditions are sufficient to bring the past back to life again, and even the pattern of moving along the wall still imitates the behavior of a former refugee.

It is important to recall that Freud for the first time described the neurotic "repetition compulsion" in relation to traumatic neurosis (Freud 1955: 18 ff.). What is meant here is the unconscious human tendency to relive or even reenact unmastered experiences of the past again and again, be it in thought, dreams, actions, games, or relationships. If, for example, the early childhood of a person is marked by abuse and violent experiences, then this motif can determine his or her later relationships in such a way that he or she unconsciously keeps creating abusive situations. This means that it is not just happy relationships that are sought or looked for, but particularly harmful and painful situations are recreated. The explanation for this lies in the unconscious fixations of body memory, which contain unfavorable patterns of perception and behavior as kinds of stage directions, tending towards their actualization even if they are no longer appropriate to external circumstances. The cyclical time structure of the unconscious overlays subsequent, similar situations and repeats an old pattern, like an old vinyl record on which the needle is stuck (Starobinski 1991: 132).

Cyclical and Linear Time

We have seen that the temporality of the body is primarily characterized by a rhythmic-periodic structure of the immediate present. Overlaying this is the long-term dynamic of cycles of deficiency, desire, and satisfaction, the rhythms of waking and sleeping, exhaustion and regeneration. Lastly, on a still larger scale, we find cyclical structure in body memory, in its habitualities and repetitions, which shape and penetrate the present either as implicit, unconscious, continued effects of the past, or which can create an immediate connection to earlier biographical experiences as a literal return of the past. Let us now consider how the linear time order develops in contrast to cyclical time.

Individual and Collective Formation of the Linear Order of Time

The cyclical time of the body is also the implicit primary temporality of the present, in which time as such is not yet conscious. The child playing obliviously does not experience explicit time. Implicit lived time is the movement of life itself and we dive into it every time we are absorbed by a perception or action, such as the "flow" experiences (Csikszentmihalyi 1991) in which the experience of time is lost in unhindered, fluid actualization. Time becomes explicit only when the past and the future as such come into view and stand out from the present. This happens primarily in the experiences of the "no longer" and "not yet" (Fuchs 2013). In the one case, something is detached from the present and slips into the *having-been*; and with this time becomes first conscious or explicit, because it "keeps going" and separates us from the lost object. Awareness of the past sharpens from early childhood on, especially with losses, separations, or disappointments. In the other case, something that we need or wish for is still to come, it is anticipated in the imagination. With the "not yet," the future as such emerges, and once again time becomes explicit, namely as a timespan of expectation or longing, that is experienced with feelings of tension, impatience, or yearning.

For a child, experiences of separation in particular are painful, worrying, or even frightening. Therefore, early socialization is characterized in all cultures by the use of rhythms, melodies, and rituals; they perform the function of giving feelings of safety, belonging, and familiarity to children through cyclical repetition and inter-bodily resonance (Fuchs & De Jaegher 2009). With the development of autobiographical memory beginning in the second year of life, the perspective of time broadens; memories of the past become possible as well as anticipations of the more distant future (Markowitsch & Welzer 2009). Gradually, one's own lifespan enters consciousness as a continuum; however, connected with this is also the knowledge of the mortality of all living things. Besides rituals, narratives now begin to perform calming and securing functions, set against the developing awareness of death: myths and fairy tales embed the present in a cyclical, recurring past or in an overarching, collective temporality, from the "once upon a time" to the "they lived happily ever after," or from the very beginning of Creation until its revelatory return to its origin. The individual lifetime, our *being-towards-death*, remains in this way embedded in natural processes and in universal time.

This imbedding is of course bound to the cyclical conceptions and organizations of time of mythical cultures and their descendants. As we have seen, the linear conception of time developed with modernity, and since then it has increasingly determined societal processes and individual consciousness. Here, I want to quickly sketch the most important causes for this development:

1) The beginning of the accumulation of capital in the Italian city states and the spreading of banking with interest (hitherto forbidden by the church) lay the bases for the long-term future-orientating of economic subjects. The capitalist principle of growth and acceleration increasingly takes the place of traditional cyclical economics (Wood 2002).

2) The introduction of public mechanical clocks from 1350 onwards licenses the rational-linear organization of time in social life in quantifiable measurements, such as in schools, or in the military, in public institutions, or in work paid according to hours instead of products.

3) Since Galileo, the scholastic idea of movement as goal- and creature-oriented is replaced in the natural sciences and technology by the principle of linear, uniform movement, which, without friction, could last indefinitely. In similar ways, at a later date, the abstract linear time of Newtonian physics replaces the cyclical conception of time of the Middle Ages.

4) Not least, the discrepancy between limited lifetime and unlimited universal world time is put into collective awareness as never before by a collective experience of death, namely the Black Death ca. 1350, to which 30–50% of the European population fell victim (Gronemeyer 1993). The individual embedding in overarching cycles of time and faith in the church as their representative begin to fade; the linear *being-towards-death* becomes irrefutable and irresolvable. This collective experience adds to the thrust of individualization as well as to a growing occupation with the here and now in the burgeoning Renaissance.

The sum of these and related developments leads to a growing decoupling of societal and economical processes from cyclical natural time. Since modernity, linear temporality is established in the collective consciousness, as well as in social and economic circumstances. However, it comes into a latent and often also manifest conflict with the cyclical time of the body and vital processes, because life does not know linear time; and one could indeed question whether death is the actual "goal" of life. Despite Freud's theory, something like the "death drive" has never been proven. Looking at it biologically, it would be nonsensical: life always strives to preserve itself in autopoietic cycles. Even though the individual is destined for death through old age or exhaustion, this may be explained as a side effect of the cyclical recurrence of life in procreation. Of course, this is just a glimpse at another aspect of temporality which cannot be discussed at depth in the present text. In whatever way death may be explained, "being-towards-death" as an existential condition is a solely human predicament.

Conflicts between Cyclical and Linear Orders of Time

The linear principle of time of Western culture stands in obvious contrast to the processes of life upon which the functioning and survival of society depend, from waking and sleeping, through metabolism, to procreation. The relation of the two orders of time remains fundamentally precarious, because, in distinction to linear processes, rhythmic cyclical processes cannot be accelerated at will. Repeatedly, we are faced with the threat of de-couplings from natural foundations and their limited (or only cyclically renewable) resources, be they of the biological environment or the individual and his body. Such de-couplings of time orders manifest themselves in ecological or economic crises, as well as in individual overexertion and illnesses.

Paul Virilio (2006) has described the constantly accelerating culture as "dromocracy," as the "rule of the race," namely the race against time. Western societies know no stoppage, no lingering, no inhibition of action; continuous activity, technical progress, economic growth, and increased consumption are the highest decrees. The symbol of time decoupling is New York, which boasts that it is "the city that never sleeps," and in whose central square, appropriately named "Times Square," never ending, flickering advertising hoardings turn night into day. The fact that the exponential increase in energy consumption cannot be reconciled with the cyclical regeneration of nature has now become obvious with global climate change. But the fundamental time conflict of industrial and post-industrial societies affects individuals equally.

The courses of time, which in the past were appropriate to the human body and processes of life, have now become unbound. The tempo of the living is replaced by the randomly increasable tempo of the inanimate, namely the data, images, and financial flows, for which distances and delays no longer exist. The explosive acceleration of traffic shrinks distances also for the human, but at the cost of the perception of the immediate environment, of *what is close*. Acceleration in time leads to a disappearance of the space in which one can rest. Unease and agitation prevail, resulting in a "determined aimlessness." Communication technologies which create a ubiquity and a simultaneity of things distant, even something like a shared universal moment, contribute to the dissolution and de-structuring of life. The result is a loss of the rhythms of life, a disturbance in the balance between the difference spheres of life, particularly between work and free time.

Against this background, let us take a look at psychopathology. Mental illnesses are also often characterized by the fact that the cyclical processes of life are derailed and the rhythmization of everyday life no longer functions (Fuchs 2001, 2013). Thus, in manic states, the movement of life accelerates and constantly overruns the cyclical time of the body and of biological diurnal rhythms, favoring instead linearly accelerated time. Manic patients ignore the needs of their body, do not grant themselves any sleep, and ignore the signs of developing exhaustion. The body is exploited mercilessly, turned into a mere vehicle and instrument of the inflated drive. The loss of the present time of the body is also manifest in the fact that manic patients only fleetingly enter into contact with the world and others, and in their restlessness, cannot tarry in the present. For them, the present is indeed determined by what is missing or what could be possible. Manics therefore live beyond their means and exhaust their biological and social resources. The rhythmic, and therefore also retarding, moment of existence is no longer perceived, but rather repressed or overrun.

On the other hand, there is the clinical picture of *depression*, which manifests not least the increasing demands placed on individuals by the accelerated processes of time in society. This includes in particular disorders that used to be termed *depressive exhaustion* (*Erschöpfungsdepression*) and nowadays are more fashionably called *burn-out syndrome*. These conditions are marked by a spiral of increasing demands upon oneself and psychophysical exhaustion. It often starts with an increasing extension of work time with the aim of satisfying external demands, avoiding social decline, or even being one of the "top performers." More and more, the structure of the day and the rhythms of exertion and recovery get lost, leading to constant strain and increasing inefficiency despite enhanced willpower, followed by dissatisfaction and frustration, inner emptiness, and exhaustion to the point of psychic decompensation (Rössler 2012). The linear principle of time here obviously exhausts psychophysical resources that are only renewable in cyclical ways. This is illustrated by a case study:

> A 34-year-old patient had started his career at a top management consultancy after graduating with brilliant grades and an MBA in the USA and had worked 60–80 hours per week. A decreasing circle of friends and a weekend partnership became a habit. For an Asian project, he commuted between the continents and allowed himself a maximum of five hours sleep per night. The shock came for him when his supervisor nevertheless certified him as having "insufficient performance".
>
> From then on, the job became a torture for the patient, and he increasingly began to doubt its meaning. Sleep disturbances, dizziness and headaches were added to this. He had the feeling that he was only functioning like a machine and only watching himself from the outside. When his girlfriend separated from him, he hardly felt any pain at all. Three weeks later he collapsed during a session and was admitted to the psychiatric clinic in suicidal condition (case study from my own practice).

The patient's life plan was characterized by a rigid performance orientation at the price of neglecting human relationships. His efforts at constant self-acceleration converged with the demands of an accelerated society but overtaxed the resources of his body. The linear principle of self-acceleration at the expense of social relations proved to be an illusion; it led to increasing emptiness, alienation, and finally to depressive breakdown.

The epidemiologically observable increase in depressive disorders in Western societies has raised the question of the extent to which depression can be understood as the typical disease of accelerated societies. Probably the best-known diagnosis of this kind was articulated by the French sociologist Alain Ehrenberg (1998/2008) with his thesis of the "exhausted self." If one follows Ehrenberg's argumentation, Freud's "discontent in culture" (*Das Unbehagen in der Kultur*) today results less from painful drive suppression than from the competitive demands of society on the subjects living in it. Depression now means capitulation to these demands of self-assertion; it becomes an epidemic of the exhausted, who regard their lagging behind others as a lack of flexibility and resilience, as an individual failure. On the other hand, they are confronted with a stratum of over-achievers who drive the manic acceleration forward in all areas of life.

Like mania, depression itself is characterized by a loss of rhythmic temporality, obviously not by acceleration but by deceleration. Depressives always complain about how slowly time passes for them, how agonizingly the day stretches out in front of them, and, in experimental studies, they tend to estimate the duration of a given time interval as longer than it really is (Bech 1975; Kitamura & Kumar 1982; Mundt et al. 1998). In addition to this, we see a disturbance of the hormonal diurnal rhythm, of the sleep-wake cycle, of drive, appetite, and interest, resulting in a loss of the cyclical-bodily structure of time that may culminate in complete lethargy, inaction, and aboulia (that is, the absence of volition). A patient from my own practice described this as follows:

> I sit at home and watch time tick away agonizingly slowly. Again a moment, again a moment. […] I am only waiting for another day to end – a pointless day, just another step on the way to my death.

This homogenized time experience in depression can also be understood as *desynchronization*, namely as a decoupling from intersubjective time (Fuchs 2001), as described by another patient of mine:

> My inner clock has stopped, while others' clocks continue to run. In everything I would have to do, I am not making any progress, I am paralyzed. I fall behind in my duties. I steal time.

Such descriptions make it clear how, in depression, time becomes a power in its own right, to which patients feel helplessly exposed. There is no doubt that depression as such is not a product of modernity—the disease of melancholy was already well known to antiquity. But, precisely as a fundamental disorder of temporality, depression, like no other mental illness, reflects the conflict between the primary, cyclical structure of life processes and the rule of linear time, which has been established in Western culture since modern times. Desynchronization, falling out of linear world time, becomes a latent threat in our competitive and accelerated society, which has to be fought against continuously. In depression, these efforts fail, the individual lags hopelessly behind, and decoupling from the common time becomes a reality.

Conclusion

We have seen that the time of living creatures is characterized at root by recurrent processes which manifest themselves in manifold ways: in the rhythmic-periodical structure of the immediate present, in longer term dynamics of deficiency, drive, satisfaction, and regeneration cycles, and finally in the repetitive structure of body memory. The temporality of implicit, bodily experience does not proceed in a linear way but rather rhythmically and cyclically, so long as this pre-reflexive experience is not superimposed by an explicit consciousness of time nor by a linear time perspective. This linear time arises with autobiographical memory, with consciousness of past and future, but ultimately with the human awareness of death, or, in Heidegger's terminology, with the "*Vorlaufen in den Tod*" (anticipation of death). In the collective consciousness, the linear principle of time has come to dominate since modern times, due to the interaction of economic, scientific, technical, and cultural conditions, and unfolds a global dynamic that continues to this day.

Cyclical and linear time stand in tension with one another, and multiple collective and individual pathologies can be traced back to a decoupling of linear dynamics from the processes of life to an acceleration and derhythmization of social or individual courses of time. This decoupling becomes particularly manifest in manic and depressive illness. Both from a psychiatric and sociopolitical point of view, it therefore seems necessary to develop strategies of retardation and inhibition and to handle the resources of the body as carefully as the resources of nature. One of the most important strategies is the *rhythmization* of life. In the treatment of burn-out and depression, for example, the restructuring of the day through periods of activity and rest is one of the basic therapeutic measures. This is because cyclical, goal-oriented temporality, which is fulfilled in the goal, counteracts the empty succession of linear time that dominates the patient. A "resynchronization therapy" (Fuchs 2019) can gradually bring the patient back into resonance with natural rhythms and common time sequences.

Rhythmizations would also be a means of inhibition against the unchecked dynamics of globalized capitalism. What would be at stake, therefore, would be resistance to the derhythmization of life, which is spreading more and more to all areas of society. For example, 24-hour opening hours or constant media accessibility are the natural enemies of cyclical bodily and thus also human time. If "time is money," then it means that the economic system as such has no inherent resistances, no built-in inhibitions that could stop the unbridled acceleration. Not only throttling measures, such as financial transaction or mobility taxes, sustainable economies, but also the systematic resistance to the quantification and homogenization of time are therefore part of the balance between cyclical and linear time, which in the long run is indispensable for an organization of society that is in accordance with life.

Similarly, the task of leading one's life consists in perennially balancing the flight of linear time with the retarding moment of cyclical, present time. This can be achieved, for example, through regularly changing between phases of acceleration and phases of retardation, or between times of striving and times of leisure and spontaneity. It can also be achieved by arcs of action which are performed in their own proper time, arriving at a destination where we can rest without already being concerned with the next occupation or distraction.

However, under current cultural conditions, the unfolding of present time increasingly requires a focused attention and practice. It is not for nothing that the meditation procedures of Asian religions revolve around the bodily present, in particular around attention to respiratory rhythm, or similarly around rhythmically habitualized activities such as recreational walking or the concentrated performance of ritual ceremonies. What is ultimately at stake is a return of consciousness from its entanglement in linear time to the *extended now*: this enables a connection to the deeper layer of body experience and body memory that is not organized in a linear sequence, but rather constantly grows through the conduct of life. On this layer of recurring bodily experience, the present may even become "extra-temporal," as Proust terms it, and in this mystical experience it may overcome the linear being-towards-death.

References

Achtner, W. et al. 1998. *Dimensionen der Zeit. Die Zeitstrukturen Gottes, der Welt und des Menschen.* Darmstadt: Wissenschaftliche Buchgesellschaft.

Appelfeld, A. 2009. *The Story of a Life: A Memoir.* New York: Random House.

Baxton, W. H., Heron, W., Scott, R. 1954 "Effects of decreased variation in the sensory environment." *Canadian Journal of Psychology* 8: 70–76.

Bech, P. 1975. "Depression: Influence on time estimation and time experience." *Acta Psychiatrica Scandinavia*, **51**: 42–50.

Bergson, H. 1988 *Matter and Memory*. **Nancy Margaret Paul** and **W. Scott Palmer** (trans.), Cambridge, MA & London: Zone Books. (Originally published 1896.)

Bergson, H. 1910. *Time and Free Will: An Essay on the Immediate Data of Consciousness.* **F. L. Pogson** (trans.), London: George Allen and Unwin (Originally Published 1889).

Bschor, T. et al. 2004. "Time experience and time judgment in major depression, mania and healthy subjects. A controlled study of 93 subjects." *Acta Psychiatrica Scandinavia* **109**: 222–229.

Craig, A. D. 2009. "Emotional moments across time: a possible neural basis for time perception in the anterior insula." *Philosophical Transactions of the Royal Society of London: Biological Sciences* B **364**: 1933–1942.

Csikszentmihalyi, M. 1991. *Flow: The Psychology of Optimal Experience*. New York: Harper Collins.

Dainton, B. 2010. "Temporal consciousness." In E. N. Zalta (ed.) *The Stanford Encyclopedia of Philosophy*, Available at: http://plato.stanford.edu/archives/fall2010/entries/consciousness-temporal (last accessed on 01/01/2021).

Eliade, M. 1959. *The Sacred and the Profane: The Nature of Religion*. **Willard R. Trask** (trans.) New York: Harcourt Brace.

Elias, N. 2007. *Time: An Essay*. Dublin: University College Dublin Press (first published in 1992 by Basil Blackwell, Oxford.)

Freud, S. 1955. "Beyond the pleasure principle." In *Standard Edition of the Works of Sigmund Freud*. Vol. **XVIII**, **James Strachey** (trans.), London: Hogarth Press (pp. 7–66).

Fuchs, T. 2001. "Melancholia as a desynchronization: Towards a psychopathology of interpersonal time." *Psychopathology* **34**: 179–186.

Fuchs, T. 2012. "The phenomenology of body memory." In S. Koch et al. (eds.) *Body Memory, Metaphor and Movement*. Amsterdam: John Benjamins (pp. 9–22).

Fuchs, T. 2013. "Temporality and psychopathology." *Phenomenology and the Cognitive Sciences* **12**: 75–104.

Fuchs, T. 2017. "Self across time: The diachronic unity of bodily existence." *Phenomenology and the Cognitive Sciences* **16**: 291–315.

Fuchs, T. 2019. "The life-world of persons with mood disorders." In G. Stanghellini, M. Broome, A. Raballo, A. V. Fernandez, P. Fusar-Poli, R. Rosfort (eds.) *The Oxford Handbook of Phenomenological Psychopathology*. Oxford: Oxford University Press, (pp. 617–633).

Fuchs, T., H. De Jaegher. 2009. "Enactive intersubjectivity: Participatory sense-making and mutual incorporation." *Phenomenology and the Cognitive Sciences*, **8**: 465–486.

Gronemeyer, M. 1993. *Das Leben als letzte Gelegenheit: Sicherheitsbedürfnisse und Zeitknappheit*, Darmstadt: Wissenschaftliche Buchgesellschaft.

Husserl, E. 1991. *On the Phenomenology of the Consciousness of Internal Time*. **John Barnett Brough** (trans.) Dordrecht: Kluwer. (Originally Published 1893.)

James, W. 1904. "Does 'consciousness' exist?" *The Journal of Philosophy* **18**: 477–491.

Jonas, H. 1966. *The Phenomenon of Life: Toward a Philosophical Biology*. New York: Harper & Row.

Kant, I. 1998. *Critique of Pure Reason*. **Paul Gruyer, Allen W. Wood** (ed. and trans.). Cambridge MA: Cambridge University Press.

Kornmeier, J., W. Ehm, H. Bigalke, M. Bach. 2007. "Discontinuous presentation of ambiguous figures: How interstimulus-interval durations affect reversal dynamics and ERPs." *Psychophysiology* **44**: 552–560.

Kitamura, T., R. Kumar. 1982. "Time passes slowly for patients with depressive state." *Acta Psychiatrica Scandinavia* **65**: 415–420.

Kiverstein, J. 2010. "Making sense of phenomenal unity: An intentionalist account of temporal experience." *Royal Institute of Philosophy Supplement* **67**: 155–181

Kjellgren, A., Lyden, F., Norlander, T. (2008). "Sensory isolation in flotation tanks: Altered states of consciousness and effects on well-being." *The Qualitative Report* **13**: 636–656.

Lévy-Bruhl, L. 1966. **Lillian A . Clare** (trans.) *How Natives Think*. New York: Washington Square Press. (Originally Published 1910.)

Lilly, J. C. 1977. *The Deep Self: Profound Relaxation and the Tank Isolation Technique*. New York: Warner Books.

London, J. 2002. "Cognitive constraints on metric systems: Some observations and hypotheses." *Music Perception* **19**: 529–550.

Malloch, S. N. 1999. "Mothers and infants and communicative musicality." *Musicae Scientiae* Special Issue 1999/2000: 9–57.

Markowitsch, H., Welzer, H. 2009. *The Development of Autobiographical Memory*. London: Psychology Press.

Meissner, K., Wittmann, M. 2011. "Body signals, cardiac awareness, and the perception of time." *Biological Psychology* **86**: 289–297.

Merleau-Ponty, M. (1962). *Phenomenology of Perception*. **Colin Smith** (trans.), London: Routledge & Kegan Paul.

Mundt, C. et al. 1998. "Zeiterleben und zeitschaetzung depressiver patienten." *Nervenarzt* **69**: 38–45.

Pollatos, O. et al. 2014. "Interoceptive focus shapes the experience of time." *PloS one* **9**(1), e86934.

Pöppel, E. 1997. "A hierarchical model of temporal perception." *Trends Cognitive Science* **1**: 56–61.

Pöppel, E. 2000. *Grenzen des Bewusstseins: Wie kommen wir zur Zeit, und wie entsteht Wirklichkeit?* Frankfurt: Insel.

Proust, M. 1992. In search of lost time. Vol. 1. In *Swann's Way*. **C. K. Scott Moncrieff, Terence Kilmartin** (trans.), New York: Random House.

Proust, M. 1993. In search of lost time. Vol. 6. In *Time Regained*. **Andreas Mayor, Terence Kilmartin** (trans.), New York: Random House.

Rössler, W. 2012. "Stress, Burnout, and Job Dissatisfaction in Mental Health Workers." *European Archives of Psychiatry and Clinical Neuroscience* **262**: 65–69.

Starobinski, J. 1991. *Kleine Geschichte des Körpergefühls*, Frankfurt: Fischer.

Stern, D. N. 2004. *The Present Moment in Psychotherapy and Everyday Life*. New York: W. W. Norton & Company.

Stern, D. N. 2010. *Forms of Vitality: Exploring Dynamic Experience in Psychology, the Arts, Psychotherapy, and Development*. Oxford: Oxford University Press.

Summa, M. 2011. "Das Leibgedächtnis. Ein Beitrag aus der Phänomenologie Husserls." *Husserl Studies* 27: 173–196.

Szelag, E., von Steinbüchel, N., Reiser, M., Gilles de Langen, E., Pöppel, E. 1996. "Temporal Constraints in processing of nonverbal rhythmic patterns." *Acta Neurobiololgical Experiments* 56: 215–225.

Virilio, P. 2006. *Speed and Politics*. Marc Polizzotti (trans.), Los Angeles: Semiotexte (Originally published 1977.)

Wittmann, M. 2009. "The inner experience of time." *Philosophical Transactions of the Royal Society of London: Biological Sciences*. B 364: 1955–1967.

Wittmann, M. 2011. "Moments in time." *Frontiers in Integrative Neuroscience* 5: 66.

Wood, E. M. 2002. *The Origin of Capitalism: A Longer View*. New York, London: Verso.

Text References (English papers)

Fuchs, T. 2014. "The virtual other. Empathy in the age of virtuality." *Journal of Consciousness Studies* **21**: 152–173.

Fuchs, T. 2020. "Embodiment and personal identity in dementia." *Medicine, Health Care and Philosophy* 23: 665–676.

Fuchs, T. 2018. "The cyclical time of the body and its relation to linear time." *Journal of Consciousness Studies* **25**: 47–65.

Index

For the benefit of digital users, indexed terms that span two pages (e.g., 52–53) may, on occasion, appear on only one of those pages.

Tables and figures are indicated by *t* and *f* following the page number.

vs. indicates a comparison